Dr Nick Fuller is a leading obesity researcher in Australia. He has worked in both corporate and academic settings and in his current position is responsible for the clinical research program at the Boden Institute, Charles Perkins Centre, at the University of Sydney. He has helped thousands of people with their weight-loss and lifestyle journeys over the past 15 years and investigated a broad range of areas, including dietary and exercise programs, appetite regulators, commercial programs, complementary and conventional medicines, medical devices and surgical treatments. He has degrees in exercise physiology, nutrition and dietetics, and a doctorate in obesity and weight management. For more information visit www.intervalweightloss.com.au or the 'Dr Nick Fuller's Interval Weight Loss' Facebook page.

Dr Nick Fuller

interval WEIGHT LOSS for Life

LIFE

PENGUIN LIFE

UK | USA | Canada | Ireland | Australia
India | New Zealand | South Africa | China

Penguin Books is part of the Penguin Random House group of companies whose addresses can be found at global.penguinrandomhouse.com.

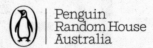

Penguin
Random House
Australia

First published in Australia by Penguin Life in 2018

Text copyright © Nicholas Fuller, 2018

Cover design by Christabella Designs
Author photograph courtesy of Ogilvy PR Health and Dan Gosse images
Printed and bound in Australia by Griffin Press, an accredited ISO AS/NZS 14001 Environmental Management Systems printer.

A catalogue record for this book is available from the National Library of Australia

NATIONAL LIBRARY OF AUSTRALIA

ISBN: 978 0 14379 107 2

penguin.com.au

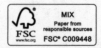

MIX
Paper from responsible sources
FSC
www.fsc.org   FSC® C009448

This book is for you, Dad.

You inspired me to always put my work into words,
and to teach and help others.

You will forever be in my thoughts and I miss you
very much.

CONTENTS

INTRODUCTION

If you're exhausted by your battle with your weight, you're not alone. I am a leading weight-loss researcher at the University of Sydney, and after 15 years working in this field I have helped countless patients from different cultures, backgrounds and age groups who have had only one thing in common: their failure to lose weight.

Although the media loves to portray those who struggle with their weight as lazy and uneducated – the implication being that it's all *their* fault – this simply isn't true. Many of my patients have been highly educated and, far from being lazy, the vast majority have been so committed to losing weight that they had tried numerous diets before they met me. How could it be, then, that they had still been gaining weight, I wondered? And why were my group of patients simply a microcosm of what was going on at a much larger scale in Australia and across the globe? Could the very act of dieting have something to do with their weight gain?

Determined to help, I made it my mission to find out. My team and I managed to make some crucial findings that really can make a difference. Certainly the vast majority of my patients went on to lose weight and keep it off long term under my guidance, using what I call the Interval Weight Loss approach.

My first book, *Interval Weight Loss*, outlined this technique, which is based on the concept of the 'set point'. Everybody has a set point – the weight your body is most comfortable being at and tries to defend when you gain or lose weight. It's the weight that you remain at for a long period of time and that you'll bounce back to after every bout of dieting you attempt. The Interval Weight Loss approach helps your body to work differently so it feels comfortable at its new weight and doesn't work to defend its set point.

After *Interval Weight Loss* was published, the response from readers was overwhelming and I received a flood of letters from people thanking me for writing the book and saying they could relate to the stories of yo-yo dieting I was sharing. Many people also requested consultations. As much as I'd like to take on lots of new private patients, it isn't feasible, but fortunately for many people it's also not necessary to be in a hospital clinic to lose weight (and nor do you require the team of specialist chefs and personal trainers that celebrities have). With the new information contained in this book, you will be empowered to succeed.

Some of you may be turning to this book because you've read *Interval Weight Loss* and are either on your way to achieving, or have achieved, your ideal body weight and want to maintain it. Some of you may have plateaued and need further tips. And some may not have read my first book and wonder what Interval Weight Loss is all about. Whatever your reason for picking up *Interval Weight Loss for Life*, I hope you find it a practical guide to sustainable weight loss that you can turn to whenever you're struggling. It's intended to be a step-by-step guide that gives further information on Interval Weight Loss and how to apply it to your own life *long term*. I'll get into the nitty gritty of the Interval Weight Loss plan so that no challenge will bring you unstuck. And since I'm glad to say many of you were kind enough to write in saying you found the recipes in my first book helpful, I have included some new meals that are nutritious, tasty and designed to be easy enough for the whole family to enjoy.

PART 1

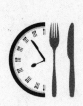

CHAPTER 1

THE SKINNY
ON WEIGHT GAIN

'We are drowning in information but starved
for knowledge' – *John Naisbitt*

Two out of every three people now struggle with excess weight. We are getting fatter as a society and this is consistent across the globe. More and more people who were previously overweight (clinically diagnosed by a Body Mass Index of 25–30 kg/m^2) have now developed obesity (a Body Mass Index of more than 30 kg/m^2) – a more concerning condition still.

The obesity rate for North American adults is currently at a whopping 38 per cent, and the United States is the heaviest nation in the world. Running a close second is its bordering neighbour, Mexico, with an obesity rate of 32 per cent, followed by New Zealand, Hungary, Australia and the United Kingdom. At an enormous obesity rate of 28 per cent, we are the world's fifth fattest people. And things are only going to get worse. It's predicted that by 2030, these numbers will hit 47 per cent for the United States, 39 per cent for Mexico and 35 per cent for Australia and the United Kingdom. It's my mission to reverse this upward trend in Australia.

Unlike Australia, countries such as the United States consider obesity a disease. In fact, the World Health Organization published a report in 2000 stating that obesity was a chronic disease that had become 'so common that it is replacing the more traditional public health concerns, including under-nutrition and infectious disease, as one of the most significant contributors to ill health'.

Why? Because it's extremely hard to return to a healthy weight from being overweight. The body is smart and will tend to work back to its starting point, or what I refer to as the 'set point' (more on this later). Yes, it's easy to lose those first few kilos, but very difficult to keep them off long term. Your body will make it difficult not to regain the weight you lose every single time. And, sadly, with this excess body weight you are more likely to develop other diseases down the track such as type 2 diabetes and heart disease, to name just a couple. Your body stops working as efficiently when it carries excess fat, because fat is a stress on the body, preventing vital organs such as the liver from doing their job properly.

Your weight can creep up without you noticing and, as

my client Jasmine discovered, there are key points in your life when you're susceptible to gaining weight.

Jasmine was a healthy 64 kg at the end of high school and with a height of 1.66 cm had a BMI of 23.2 kg/m². But as she moved into the workforce, she drank more wine, moved less and went out for dinner too much. She found herself ballooning to 72 kg, just 10 years later, at the age of 28. This is a common scenario as an increase in weight often coincides with a change in life stage such as going to university, getting married, having children or starting a new job.

When Jasmine realised how much weight she had put on, she did what many of you will also have done: turned to the internet for advice. And guess what happened? Yes, you've got it! She put on even more weight.

The scientist versus the celebrity

We live in a society where we are bombarded with misleading and conflicting information when it comes to nutrition and weight loss, predominantly by unqualified social media sensations, YouTubers and TV celebrities. With health and wellness being so central to our long-term survival, why do we trust advice from celebrities who are being paid to fake their way through it? The population has been brainwashed by weight-loss propaganda for decades, and the very people we should be listening to – namely, academics and researchers – often struggle to articulate their research papers beyond an academic and clinical setting. It's a strange paradox that often the people with the best brains are completely ineffective when it comes to communicating a concept. They are brilliant thinkers, but hopeless marketers! For diets or weight-loss programs that are developed in the lab this means that the concept fails to escape the lab itself, leaving the media messaging to celebrities and marketing gurus.

My objective, therefore, is to be an academic who breaks the trend, and takes vital information about weight loss beyond a hospital and lab setting, so that I can help not just the morbidly obese, but people like Jasmine who have steadily been gaining weight. I want everyone to have the facts, and am determined to broadcast them as far and wide as I can via this book, via television, via media and social media, so that the scourge of obesity and fake diets is finally unpicked at the seams.

I have been lucky enough to complete three university degrees covering nutrition, diets, metabolism, exercise physiology, and a doctorate in obesity treatment. I have helped people at a ground level and examined what happens within their bodies from both a physiological and psychological perspective. I am passionate about helping people, and have worked one on one with patients – thousands of unhappy and often desperate people. My aim has always been to assist through learning, and to help get people's lives back on track, to give them real answers and solutions.

The Interval Weight Loss (IWL) plan is a program based on scientific research, and is designed not simply to help you lose the weight – because anyone can lose weight – but to also try to help you maintain that weight loss long term. For those interested in the science, the latest research in this field can be accessed via the 'Dr Nick Fuller's Interval Weight Loss' Facebook page.

Why is the Interval Weight Loss plan different from the latest celebrity diet?

IWL is NOT a theory, NOT a fad, NOT the latest craze. Nor is it a celebrity program based on anecdata or testimonials. It is a scientific method that is based on years of clinical and academic research. Fundamental to IWL is the universal notion of the 'set point'. Our bodies are much smarter than we think. They are fine-tuned machines that are calibrated to prevent any disturbance in equilibrium. The IWL plan taps into your body's evolutionary desire to take it back to its natural preferred weight – its optimal weight – which allows it to be efficient for its day-to-day activities.

Imagine that within your body is a silhouette of what your body should be: your optimum weight. After years of stress on the body through dieting, we need to rediscover this silhouette of you (or discover it for the first time) by following the IWL plan. This applies to EVERYONE – you can be tall, short, male, female and any cultural heritage, it doesn't matter. IWL taps deep into your body's physiology and is therefore applicable to all. The capacity for change is already within you.

Food 'experts'

A common misconception, regularly repeated by the media, is that particular nutrients or foods are to blame. There are anti-fat, anti-carbohydrate and anti-protein brigades. With social media at our fingertips, everyone, it seems, is a food expert these days. But food must be looked at from a holistic perspective. Despite what you may have read, been told, or seen on TV, no single food is to blame for the obesity epidemic or your growing waistline. And food processing and agricultural development aren't the culprits either, though our sensationalist media loves to point the finger at them.

The appeal of the quick fix

We have to consider our own role in our problems. In our modern time-poor environment the last thing on our 'to do' list is often our health, meaning it doesn't get ticked off EVER. Then we all prick up our ears when we hear about the next diet that's hit the shelves, or the new program that has been brought out by a TV celebrity or social media influencer. Because if they're a celebrity and we know who they are, they must have all the answers, right? These celebrities on Instagram simply don't know what they are talking about and their advice is not evidence-based. We are a population looking for the 'quick fix' or the 'magic bullet', but such a thing never has and never will exist.

Body image and negative food culture

The problem is also cultivated by our perception of what we believe (or, more importantly, what we have been led to believe) is a healthy body image. There has been a shift in our notion of what this ideal weight and body image is, and as a result we create an unrealistic and unhealthy goal. The prevalence of social media means that we can now look at these self-proclaimed 'experts' all the time – they are in the palms of our hands 24/7, from all over the world. It's insidious and puts doubt in our mind about how we look and what is normal. When we look at ourselves in the mirror every day, we convince ourselves that we are fat and think, 'Maybe I'll try that diet if I'll look like them.' But social media is for fantasy, NOT advice. That ripped guy or pretty girl on Instagram spruiking skinny tea or waist trainers is only setting you up for failure.

How much weight do you really need to lose?

It's all too common for people who have never had a significant weight problem to try to lose more weight than they need to, or for those who only want to lose a couple of kilos for a special occasion to take drastic measures, and in so doing trigger the perpetual cycle of dieting followed by bingeing.

A client of mine, Rachel, first presented to me with concerns about her body weight. When she first attended the clinic she had recently started a low-carb diet. Weighing in at 69 kg and 165 cm tall this meant her BMI was only 25.3 kg/m^2, but her waist circumference was just above the recommended 80 cm cut-off, at 81 cm, which suggested a slightly increased risk of heart disease and stroke. After taking her clinical history, I advised her to stop the diet and make some slight changes to her lifestyle and to not focus on her body weight, since that was healthy. Unfortunately, Rachel was too fixated on an upcoming wedding that she was to be a bridesmaid for to heed my advice, and decided to continue the low-carb diet. She lost the 5 kg she wanted to, but returned to the clinic 10 months later only to complain that she was 8 kg heavier than when I had first met her. She had been on three diets during this time, had been to two weddings and an engagement party, only to lose and regain more weight each time.

Sadly, Rachel's metabolism had also slowed during this period because of the dieting stress she had imposed on her body. I'm glad to say Rachel eventually put the principles of Interval Weight Loss into place and managed to get back down to 69 kg. Her waist circumference is now 78 cm seven years later, but it could have been so much easier had she not embarked on those crash diets in the first place, not to mention healthier.

On average, people take drastic measures four to five times a year, promising themselves that the new 'health kick' or diet they are on will be the lasting change they are looking for. A recent poll in Britain showed that a female by the age of 45 years will have tried 61 diets, and over their entire lifespan will have spent 31 years dieting. That is absolute insanity!

Cultural obsession

Our continual focus on losing weight has become a cultural norm. New diets are constantly emerging and we try each and every one of them. As we all know, you can't stick to them for very long and sadly you see a reversion to old ways and the reintroduction of those unhealthy life-style habits. We have been taught to believe that diets are the answer, but going on the next diet that hits the shelves will only make your problem worse. Your body learns to save a little extra in storage for that next bout of starvation you will put it through (it's evolutionarily ingrained in human beings), and you often end up fatter and more discouraged than before you started.

Celebrities

There are all sorts of problems with diets and weight-loss programs. The most alarming issue is that they are brought out by unqualified people who have no idea what they are talking about. The same goes for those reality TV weight-loss programs. Keep-fit fanatics and finan-cially incentivised celebrity chefs are the very last people who should be advising us on how we should eat or what we should do to shift those kilos. Obesity is a serious problem – a disease – and should not be the focus of a reality show intended for voyeuristic pleasure. Can you imagine screening a reality TV show centred on cancer patients? It's a horrifying thought, so why do we subject those with morbid obesity to it?

Every time a celebrity brings out a new product or book, we cling to the hope that this will be the answer to our weight problems and our unhappiness, despite the fact that we have failed on all the previous programs. Just because they are in the spotlight and media every day of the week doesn't mean we should listen to them. And, yes, this includes all those names that have dominated the industry for a very long time. You know who they are! They're the ones telling you that you can change your body in 12 weeks, or that eating like a caveman will somehow miraculously improve your wellbeing. They're the very people we have been buying products from for many years.

The simple truth is that most people can't stick to diets. The vast majority of diets have been brought out since the 1980s, yet we have become fatter since then. The only reason some of them stick around is because they are backed by big business or celebrities/influencers plugging them every day of the week. They are the ones making money, and sadly it's at the expense of your health and peace of mind.

The one-percenters

You will always have the one-percenters who succeed on a particular diet or plan, but this doesn't mean the diet works. Individual responses to diets vary enormously, and although people won't hesitate to tell you of their short-term success, regrettably they are not still bragging of their success five years down the track. The ketogenic (keto) diet (one of the latest fads) was ranked the worst diet for your health in 2018 in the *U.S. News and World Report*, which reviews the latest diets every year with respect to their science, specifically focusing on nutritional balance, health benefits, ease of following, safety and, of course, weight loss. Surprisingly to some, other popular diets in 2018 were also ranked among the worst and appeared in the bottom 10. These included the Dukan diet, the fast (5:2) diet, the hormone diet and the Paleo diet.

The problem with dieting

There are two main reasons why diets don't work:

1. They are unrealistic and unsustainable, requiring us to omit certain foods or even entire food groups. We are unable to stick to them for very long and after we come off the diet or program we reintroduce the foods, go back to our old ways, and stack the weight back on. Worryingly, a lot of these diets are very dangerous for our long-term health. Examples include the Paleo diet, the keto diet, or any form of low-carbohydrate diet that contains a very high intake of meat and low amount of wholegrain

carbohydrate. A high intake of meat is associated with cancer, as is a low intake of wholegrains. These eating habits are certainly not part of a healthy, balanced diet.

2. We are all tuned to a 'set point' and absolutely NO diets or weight-loss programs (whatever you want to call them, they are all achieving the same thing) address the 'set point'.

Celebrity diets/weight-loss programs

The worst thing you can do when you next commit to losing weight is to go on any new diet that hits the shelves, or that your family, friends or work colleagues tell you about. Scientific research into the 'set point' has proven that they DON'T work. Some celebrities have even acknowledged that there is a propensity to put weight back on after going on their diets, and changed their marketing angle accordingly to home in on preventing weight regain. This sounds like good and progressive change, but in truth these are only slightly altered diet ideas and yet more marketing spin, and they lack the necessary research to prove their worth and effectiveness.

And it's not just this change to a focus on preventing weight regain we are seeing. It seems that celebrities will market anything to capture the attention of their followers, shifting their stance whenever they have a new book to sell. I could write all day about the numerous flaws and health concerns with these diets, but you will find all this in my first book. Simply put, science has disproved them.

Enough is enough – the industry has been in need of disruption for a very long time. The problem has only escalated as more and more celebrities have jumped on the wellness and weight-loss bandwagon to capitalise on this lucrative US$60 billion industry, with everything from diets, to diet pills, to fancy gym memberships, to meal plans and delivery of food. There are new products on the market every week – and the more we spend the fatter we become!

What is the set point?

The set point is the weight at which we are most comfortable and it's the weight that you will remember being at for a long period of time in your adult years. Our body protects the set point whenever you impose a stress upon it. Your body doesn't like the equilibrium being altered and will minimise any disturbance. In the case of dieting, the body will want to work back to its set point, otherwise known as your starting weight. Unfortunately, this means you are in for a battle every time you start a diet. Your body ensures this!

You might be wondering, how does it protect the set point? The body is very clever and it defends us in times of stress. Dieting is one of the biggest stresses you can impose on the body. Essentially, whenever weight loss occurs through a reduction in calories, you will experience a drop in metabolism (how much energy you burn at rest) and a change in appetite hormones (telling you to eat more), and these two main changes ensure you work back to your set point. But to make matters worse, your metabolism doesn't recover and your appetite hormones keep telling you to eat more even after you regain the weight, so you may end up heavier than before. You could end up worse off for going on the diet! This is your body's attempt to survive famine (starvation). Unfortunately, our bodies are too smart for our own good and will try to make you go back to where you started – your set point – by lowering your metabolism and making you hungrier.

How is Interval Weight Loss different?

I wrote *Interval Weight Loss* to clear up all the misleading and confusing information that we are told every day of the week in relation to health and diet, and to teach people how to actually go about losing weight. I wanted to instil a passion for food that readers may never have known existed, allowing people to lose weight in a fun and easy way. And I'm not talking about the type of fun where you have to count calories, can only eat carrot and celery sticks, have to rely on meal replacements, or eliminate all forms of carbohydrate to shed the kilos. In fact, this plan is the complete opposite.

The one thing I do insist is that you're patient. Remember, this is not an approach that results in overnight success. It should, however, result in health and achieving your long-term weight-loss goals, which is undoubtedly a good trade-off.

What is the Interval Weight Loss plan?

IWL is not a diet, nor is it temporary. It is a meaningful way of changing your life for the better that involves:

• A month-on, month-off plan following the food and exercise principles that are intended to recalibrate your body's set point so you can actually reach your body's optimum weight and stay there. For example, during a weight-loss month, you need to monitor your lifestyle closely by planning your food intake and prioritising exercise, to lose up to 2 kg per month. In the weight-maintenance month that follows, you can relax and enjoy more treats and takeaway as a way of ensuring you don't lose any more weight and to help the body to get used to its new set point.

- An increase in the consumption of wholesome, nutritious foods that are filling and tasty, allowing you to eat more than you're used to.
- The freedom to relax and enjoy treats or takeaway food more frequently in weight-maintenance months to ensure you stay at your new weight and don't lose an unsustainable amount in a short period of time, and to enable the body to get used to its new set point.
- Exercise that you enjoy but can fit within the constraints of your lifestyle.
- The flexibility to customise the plan to fit your lifestyle choices and include dietary restrictions, for example, vegetarianism, coeliac disease, type 2 diabetes or dairy intolerance.
- A fully supported online community found at 'Dr Nick Fuller's Interval Weight Loss' Facebook page.

It does not involve:
- Calorie counting or following set meal plans.
- Weighing out portions of foods for each meal.
- Complex cooking that requires you to track down an abundance of ingredients for each meal.
- Locating obscure ingredients in supermarkets or health food stores.
- Adopting an exercise or activity routine that is not sustainable or enjoyable.

Am I destined to fail if I have dieted all my life?

No, absolutely not! Many of us are imprisoned by the constant cycle of feast or famine, the never-ending dieting cycle that we have imposed on ourselves. It's time to break that cycle! The IWL plan can be followed by anyone and with any amount of weight to lose, from a few kilos to 50!

Is it too late to start the Interval Weight Loss plan?

The earlier you put the principles of the IWL lifestyle into action, the easier it is, but I believe anyone can reprogram their set point into a new set point – a lower body weight that the body thrives at. Those who have more weight to lose just need to follow the plan for longer. Our bodies are stubborn and the stress we have imposed on them (for example, eating poorly, exercising little and neglecting sleep) has seen our set points or baseline weight go up over time. If the body is put under stress over a significant period, something has to give.

On average there is an increase in body weight of approximately 0.5–1.0 kg for every year from early adulthood through to middle age. Preventing your set point going up, of course, makes it easier to get back to a healthy body weight.

It is always easier to kick the kilos early to prevent your set point going up, but you will still succeed on the IWL plan regardless of your current weight.

Over the next chapters you will learn:

- The psychology of adapting to success
- How to calculate your set point
- What and how much to eat
- How to exercise
- How to organise and get the most out of your day
- How to prevent those bouts of comfort or emotional eating that are all too common.

It's never too late, so read on to find out how to get started. And if you get stuck at any point along the way you can ask questions through the Interval Weight Loss website and Facebook page.

CHAPTER 2

THE FIRST STEP

'A journey of a thousand miles begins with a
single step' – *Lao-Tzu*

The psychology of adapting to success is the very first
step. Many people have unrealistic expectations about
the speed, ease and consequences of changing a behaviour.
I call this 'false hope syndrome'. Actual change takes time,
effort and patience, but it is not a linear process and it is
normal to take a backward step at times. In fact, it takes
66 days to create a new habit or to break an old one. Yes,
that's right, it takes more than two months before a new
behaviour becomes automatic. The brain acts in a similar
way to a muscle that is repeatedly used and strengthened
over time, so perseverance is the only way to successfully
break through the wall.

The hijacking of our brains

There is a reason it's so hard to resist foods we love. When we register a pleasure, dopamine is released into the brain's pleasure centre, called the nucleus accumbens. The hippocampus is then responsible for remembering this sense of satisfaction and the amygdala triggers a response next time we see the food, almost as if our brains have been hijacked.

Nature's treats

Since the industrial revolution and the shift to mass production, the foods that give us pleasure are no longer nature's treats, such as papaya, mangoes and berries, but rather processed foods. The added fat, salt and sugars in these manufactured foods trigger addictive-like eating behaviours, which we see reflected in our modern obsession with foods such as Freak Shakes, doughnuts, muffins, McDonald's, Pizza Hut and Nutella. (The latter even caused fights to break out in supermarkets in France when Nutella was sold briefly at a steep discount.) These foods are convenient, taste good and are hard to avoid, but processed foods should not be part of your *daily* eating plan – and they're certainly nothing to fight about!

The tribal influence

Humans are tribal and seek the behaviours in others that validate their own status within the tribe. Charles Darwin wrote about this as far back as 1871 in *The Descent of Man*. It's always fascinated me that the vast majority of my patients describe their immediate family and friends as being of a similar weight category to them. This introduces a challenge. As an individual your ability to keep your goals on track is highly influenced by those closest to you. Often, patients who are committed to the program when they are in the clinic, find it harder when they get home and succumb to the influence of loved ones. For example, a cake is on the table and the family is eating the cake. How do you say no to a slice when you would previously always say yes? As a tribal society, people are made uncomfortable by those breaking the mould. Even though your decision to decline that slice of cake will be difficult, because you are breaking from that tribal mould, it is the choice that you need to make if you are to lose weight and improve your health.

A major step to adapting to success is making that very first positive choice. Applied repeatedly over time, positive decision-making becomes a wiring – the connectivity between the neurons in your brain – that is worked and strengthened. I just gave the example of the cake but it could just as easily be a weekly outing to the pub with colleagues or friends, and learning to say NO to those chips or snacks as your friend heads to the bar. This first step is most important. Repeatedly applying correct choices will lead to success.

Brain 'plasticity'

For many, dieting success lies within the architecture of their brain. Our brain structure can change over time and a lifetime of poor food choices based on processed and addictive foods may mean you find it harder to change your eating habits and re-wire your brain so that healthy food choices become the default option. But the good news is you can change the architecture of your brain and it does respond to new situations, environments and lifestyles.

Research has shown that the grey matter volume in the prefrontal cortex – the part of the brain that makes decisions – determines a person's ability to restrain themselves or implement self-control when it comes to food choices. But this research doesn't mean some people now have a scapegoat to blame for their eating habits – it means we know more about how the brain works!

Healthy eating patterns have been shown to be associated with increased brain volume and less age-related shrinkage. If you can consistently promote self-control, you can change your brain structure, increasing the connectivity of neurons, and, over time, healthier food choices become easier. So the good news is you can improve your ability to exercise self-control over what you eat, but it won't happen overnight and cutting processed and addictive foods out altogether is not the answer!

Saying no to that cake or those chips doesn't mean you can never have them but it does mean you need to be able to say no the *majority* of the time. Nowadays we are presented with these foods most days – they have become more than an occasional indulgence at a birthday or celebration. Our bodies are not designed to eat these type of foods daily and if we have too many of them we become addicted.

I can provide you with the right information and guidance to help you break free from this addiction, but you still need to be open to change. Once you've read this book it's then over to you to have an open mind and adopt a positive attitude to change, to ensure you take the necessary steps to break the cycle. I always say that your mind is like a sponge: it absorbs whatever it is surrounded by, so it is best that you keep it far away from pollutants. The wrong knowledge is a pollutant. The right knowledge cleanses.

CHAPTER 3

RESETTING
YOUR SET POINT

'All things are difficult before they are easy' –
Thomas Fuller

In the first chapter I discussed how diets are doing us harm.
I also discussed the concept of our 'set point' and how
the body will always protect its set point or level of fatness
with each diet you attempt. Years of dieting can cause
much stress on the body, including a severely compromised
metabolism (i.e. how much energy you burn at rest) and
an unfavourable change in your appetite hormones (those
signals being sent from your stomach to your brain telling
you to eat more). As a result, your body doesn't work as
well as it used to before the diet escapade. Just look at the
contestants who have appeared on *The Biggest Loser*. Down
the track from the show, not only have they regained all

the weight they lost, their metabolisms are slower than ever before – meaning they burn less energy at rest, which in turn means they have to work harder to burn food. This is a VERY bad situation to be in because we rely on our metabolism to help keep the weight off. Coupled with this slower metabolism, our appetite hormones remain altered after regaining the weight and we keep getting signals to our brain telling us to eat more.

The wash-out period

A wash-out period is particularly important before starting the IWL plan if you have had an extensive history of dieting, have recently come off a diet, or are currently on a diet. When I refer to a wash-out period I mean a period where you DON'T weigh yourself or worry at all about what happens to your weight, though you must start to follow the food plan outlined in this book. The idea is to introduce the concepts of IWL that teach you to eat when you are hungry, to nourish your body with good food and to become aware of feelings of fullness. You cannot expect to switch from a fad weight-loss program to the IWL plan and get the results that you want straight away. You simply won't!

If you are currently following a diet, stop immediately. If you have recently finished a diet and have not yet regained all the weight you lost, you will most likely have to wait until your body fights back to its set point. I'm not going to sugar-coat it: I'm afraid that it could take months, depending on how much weight you lost and how drastic a measure you took. But the good news is you can still put all of the principles of the IWL plan into place. You just need to wait before you see the weight-loss results and shouldn't expect to lose weight from the outset (more on this shortly). Remember, though, that it CAN eventually be reversed and by taking the focus off your weight you will experience a greater quality of life and psychological improvements in your lifestyle as soon as you start implementing the IWL plan. You will also allow your body to *recover* from the stress recently imposed on it.

A client of mine, Sam, had been dieting all his life before coming to see me. He had tried every diet under the sun and had seen an increase in his weight of about 1 kg each year for the past 12 years. Sam had just finished the '5:2/fast diet' and had not yet regained all of the 6 kg from his recent dieting attempt. He was still on the rebound and had put on 4 kg, so I explained the scenario his body was reacting to. It was agreed that he would introduce all the foods from the Interval Weight Loss plan into his diet and that he would not worry about his weight. However, when Sam started to see an increase on the scales immediately after I told him to reintroduce grains and fruit, he panicked. This wasn't true weight gain (as I'll explain later) but rather because his body water content was increasing from the amount of carbohydrate in these foods.

It took a month before Sam was able to stop weighing himself, which was very good considering he had been weighing himself every day and sometimes three times a day for the last 20 years. After three months of eating and enjoying the food on the Interval Weight Loss plan (a period I knew was sufficient for Sam to have regained all of the weight he had lost on the diet and stabilise his set point), we then reintroduced the idea of weighing – but only once per week. We recorded and plotted Sam's weight each week and monitored the trend over time. We also made some small changes to the type of activity he was doing to trigger a weight-loss phase. To Sam's surprise, his weight started to decrease with this new lifestyle and plan, at a rate of approximately 0.5 kg per week. Sam went on to lose 15 kg over 15 months and has been able to continue with the Interval Weight Loss plan ever since. Five years later Sam has not only kept off the 15 kg but has also been able to achieve a further 5 kg weight loss in the last six months, meaning he is 20 kg lighter. He is healthy and less fearful of putting on weight.

Reintroducing foods

Reflect back on Chapter 1 and the two main reasons diets fail. The first reason was because of their unrealistic and unhealthy nature. More often than not a diet will require us to omit certain foods or food groups. A commonly asked question raised by people first starting the IWL plan is 'Why do I see a weight change on the scales when particular foods are reintroduced?' The most common reason, as Sam found, is because of carbohydrates. Carbs are a common scapegoat for all our weight problems, but all you are experiencing when you add carbs to your daily intake is an increase in water content in the body. Carbs are made up of many sugar units which can be bundled together and stored as glycogen in the body. As it turns out, each gram of glycogen binds 3 grams of water. That ends up weighing quite a bit but is no reason for concern.

While the number on the scales might have gone up, this is not an increase in fat mass but rather an increase in water content in the body. People see this change on the scales and panic, as Sam did. They assume it must be true weight gain after reintroducing carbohydrates in meals. But in actual fact, carbs are going to help you lose the weight and you're only noticing an increase in fluid. By including a wash-out period of at least one month to ensure your weight stabilises, you will come to terms with this adjustment and not jump to the wrong conclusion.

All too often I hear clients tell me they are still avoiding particular foods and putting aspects of what they refer to as a 'low-carb' diet into place when I first see them. As a result they fear pasta and grains, believing they cause weight gain. Many of them are also under the impression that some fruits are 'fattening', as they have been told or read that they are high in sugar content. Of course, all of this is nonsense but it takes time for people to trust and understand how the body reacts to certain food intake.

It's important to include plenty of wholegrain carbohydrate sources as part of the IWL plan. These are the foods that are also likely to help prevent lifestyle diseases such as certain types of cancer, type 2 diabetes and heart disease. So, if you have been following a low-carb diet and then have suddenly switched to the IWL plan, don't be disheartened when you see the number on the scales go up with the reintroduction of healthy wholegrain carbohydrates. It's just water!

How do I know what my set point is?

Can you remember a weight you were at for a long period – say, for one year – in the past five years? This is likely to be a weight you have always hovered around – your set point. Once you have reached that weight and your body weight is stable, you are at your usual set point and can realistically expect to see weight-loss results on the IWL plan. For some, your current weight may be your set point if you have been at that weight for a year or more, even if that's the heaviest you have been.

What if I haven't weighed myself regularly over the past five years?

If you haven't weighed yourself very often in recent years, there is no need for concern. Perhaps your scales have broken, or you just couldn't face seeing the number on the dial. That's okay! This is most likely a good thing as it suggests you haven't been dieting. Just go out and find a *reasonable-quality* set of scales (I know it's tempting to rush out and get the cheapest but they'll only return unreliable measures) and see what weight you're at now. You can do it! It's only a number! And think of how great you'll feel when you see that number go down over time.

Begin by weighing yourself weekly for a month while introducing the Interval Weight Loss plan and observe the trend in your weight. If it stays stable and your clothes have been fitting the same for at least a year, you are most likely at your set point and ready to implement a weight-loss month on the IWL plan.

Are there exceptions to the wash-out rule?

There are exceptions. If you are confident that you are currently at your set point and perhaps don't have an extensive history of dieting, you will see success on the IWL plan from the get-go. If you don't lose weight straight away, it's no need for concern. The IWL plan will work ultimately but you need to shift your mindset from the quick fix that we have become dependent on. Stay committed and focus on making a great future.

General rule of thumb

Even if you have recently been on a diet and regained all the weight you lost, it doesn't hurt to start by following a wash-out period and a month of weight maintenance on the IWL plan before attempting to kick off a weight-loss month, just to make sure your body has re-calibrated to its set point. I cannot repeat this enough: you MUST ensure your weight has stabilised before starting out on a weight-loss month. And don't expect to lose weight straight away if you have been a long-term chronic dieter. It may take months for your body to kick into a weight-loss phase. Don't worry, though, as I will give you some tips for over-coming this and for speeding things up. It may seem like a drawn-out process but it will ensure you never have to diet again. Isn't that worth it?

CHAPTER 4

IDEALISM
AND REALISM

'The pessimist complains about the wind;
the optimist expects it to change; the realist
adjusts the sails' – *William Arthur Ward*

Genetics are not to blame for the increasing prevalence of obesity. You can lose weight just as effectively as the next person regardless of your genes. Remember, this is the underlying concept of IWL – anyone can follow it and anyone can succeed on it – but there are certain things to take into consideration when determining your weight-loss goal. Defining a realistic and achievable new 'set point' is the first step towards success on the IWL plan.

Calculating your goal set point

Write down your set point on the *top* of a large palm card – this is your current body weight after following the steps in Chapter 3 to ensure you are at your set point. Everyone's is different.

To give you an example: *Petra's body weight was 80 kg 20 years ago but is now 95 kg, the heaviest weight she has been. Since Petra has remained at 95 kg for some months, her set point is NOT 80 kg, it is 95 kg. This is the weight (95 kg) Petra would need to write down as it is the weight her body is defending.*

Now I want you to write down on the same palm card, on the *bottom* section, the lowest body weight you have been in your adult years. In the example provided, Petra's was 80 kg at the age of 25 years.

Petra shouldn't aim initially to get to 80 kg. Instead, she should choose a new set point that is in between her lowest weight as an adult and her current set point. *A good starting point for Petra would be 87 kg or a weight loss of approximately 8 kg. She may then be able to lose more (say, 10, 15 or even 20 kg) if she doesn't have an extensive history of dieting which has imposed damage on her body.*

If you don't want to work this out for yourself, you can make contact through the 'Dr Nick Fuller's Interval Weight Loss' Facebook page for guidance on a goal weight loss that is individually achievable for you.

You need to start with a realistic goal and then reassess

this goal *after* you achieve it – you won't get there any slower by doing this. Write the new goal set point in big letters in the *middle* of the palm card. *Petra would write down 87 kg.* This will be your reference point at all times and should be placed in a visible spot where you can always see it.

Write it down

Once you have worked out your current set point and your goal set point you are ready to start the IWL plan. Make a few different palm cards with your current set point, your new goal set point and your goal weight loss on them and place these cards in various places where they will be visible to you every day after you wake up, such as your desk or in your wallet. It is important to visualise this goal and to focus on the long term.

What other indicators can I use?

Body Mass Index (BMI) is used in a clinical setting to calculate whether a person is in a healthy body weight range. A healthy BMI is between 18.5 and 24.9 kg/m^2. BMI is calculated as your weight over your height squared. So, for someone who is 180 cm tall and weighs 100 kg, their BMI is 30.9 kg/m^2 (calculated as $100/(1.8 \times 1.8^2) = 100/3.24 = 30.86$). Don't worry if this is making your head spin or giving you flashbacks to your nightmare maths class! You can easily find BMI conversions online which do all the work for you so you can accurately work out what yours is and if it sits within a healthy range. A useful online calculator is available at the government website Health Direct: www.healthdirect.gov.au/bmi-calculator.

Waist circumference is another useful tool that complements BMI for a better picture of your risk of metabolic disease. For males a healthy waist girth is 78–94 cm, and for females 64–80 cm. Again, the government website Health Direct has a useful online calculator to calculate your waist circumference. There is more on this measure that you can use in your own home in Chapter 14.

What is considered a success?

Both BMI and waist circumference are great guides to assess your current health status but they do not define success.

Success is defined as a weight loss that you can achieve and maintain forever. In selecting your goal it is important to consider what a healthy and realistic body image actually is. As I've said, social media, reality TV shows and fad magazines have created a very unhealthy portrayal of an ideal body weight. Everyone is a so-called lifestyle and weight-loss expert on social media these days, and the filtered Instagram photos with accompanying Oprah empowering-style language can be misleading. The implicit message they are sending is: 'Follow me, mirror my life and you will look like me.' But this is not achievable, and just because someone is on social media with millions of followers doesn't mean they can be trusted. The same can be said of those 'before and after' weight-loss stories that you read about in magazines, proclaiming 'I LOST 45 KILOS IN 12 WEEKS!' They are not realistic and not healthy. And sadly, as you know, the people in these stories will only end up putting the weight back on after they come off the diet – though they will never tell you this. Everyone's body shape is different, and it is not helpful to try to look like those you follow on social media. In fact, it can be downright dangerous.

Stay focused on you

Despite the noise on Instagram and Facebook, you need to stay focused on your individual goals and a sustainable weight-loss plan for yourself. You need to look at yourself in the mirror and say, 'If I can lose 5 kg and keep that off forever, that is a huge success, and will significantly reduce my chance of developing lifestyle diseases associated with carrying too much weight. It will also result in me feeling more energetic, having more vitality, and having a better quality of life.'

Say something positive

Every day you should wake up and say something positive to yourself in the mirror. Be proud of what you have achieved and what you will achieve in the years to come with an improved health and lifestyle. Whether you need to lose 10 kg, 20 kg, 30 kg, 40 kg, or even 50 kg, do not compare yourself to other people as that is not healthy or realistic.

The focus must shift away from the short term (for example, the crazy diet that will see you drop two dress sizes or two belt buckle sizes in three weeks). You know that doesn't work. Beyond your lived experience, science has also proven that the short term doesn't work. This is not a six-week, eight-week, ten-week or three-month program. IWL is a way of life!

Your goal weight loss per month

When you impose a stress on the body (as with dieting), a physiological process within the body known as adaptive thermogenesis starts to take place, whereby the body's metabolism slows down to counteract the weight loss. This process can start to occur as quickly as after a 2–2.5 kg or 3 per cent weight loss, which is the weight loss that we consider clinically significant. A 3 per cent weight loss is when your body starts to work differently. The way the IWL plan works is to prevent the body's usual response to weight loss. Even though it is an individualised approach and will depend on an individual's weight-loss history and medical history, the general rule of thumb is to stick to a 2 kg weight loss over the course of a month (approximately

0.5 kg weight loss per week) to safely ensure you prevent the usual physiological responses. It is then crucial to maintain that 2 kg weight loss for the second month (i.e. to stay at the same weight for the second month) before going on to lose weight again during the third month, and so on, until your goal weight loss is achieved. This generally means no more than a 12 kg weight loss over the course of 12 months.

If you continue to lose weight during the weight-maintenance months, the IWL plan becomes just another diet to your body and you will get the same response that you have got every other time: your metabolism will drop and your body will stop working as efficiently. Your appetite hormones will also change to tell you to eat more. Namely, ghrelin, one of our hunger hormones, will go up to ensure you eat more food and regain the weight you've lost. So, you will just end up back where you started. The same applies if you lose more than the clinically significant amount of weight loss per month – you will also struggle because the same innate physiological responses will kick in.

You are most likely reading this thinking, gosh this is going to be a long journey! Yes, it is a slow and steady approach, but it's easy, fun and realistic. It becomes a way of life. Remember, anyone can lose 10 kg in four weeks or 20 kg in three months. But they cannot keep it off.

Everyone knows somebody – most likely multiple some-bodies – who has done the latest and greatest diet, only to end up a size bigger than they originally were. The IWL plan requires patience, and will challenge those who are looking for instant results. Focus on never having to diet again; no more obscure ingredients for strange recipes that leave you starving; no more staring longingly at a piece of fruit or a piece of chocolate because you've cut out sugar only to binge on McDonald's on the way home; no more hating how you feel when you fail – because you will.

Later chapters will provide you with all the methods and tips you can use if you are failing to achieve weight loss or if you are struggling to maintain your weight during a weight-maintenance month. The structured weekly plans also provide examples of what to do each month to ensure you get the best success from this new way of life. Remember, it is much better to be patient, follow this plan closely, and then never have to worry about your weight again.

CHAPTER 5

TRACKING YOUR BODY WEIGHT

'Know thyself' – *Socrates*

A key part of your success on the IWL plan relates to tracking your body weight so that you can make the small but often necessary adjustments to achieve your goal set point. It's important, therefore, that you have a good set of scales. Those that allow you to track your body weight digitally are very practical as they automatically upload your data into an app using wi-fi connectivity. Another good method, however, is to use a spreadsheet to track your weight (an example is available for free download at www.intervalweightloss.com.au). You must be able to analyse your weight data visually to watch the trend over time. It's pointless simply weighing yourself and saying you will remember the number next week, as all too often we forget. It is also a waste of time just writing your weight down on a piece of paper each week, unless it is visually plotted on a graph. By observing the trend over time – week by week – you can actually determine whether you are losing weight and dropping fat.

Self-weighing

You need to commit to weighing yourself frequently. This should be done once per week so that you can watch the trend in body weight over time. When you first start the IWL plan you can weigh yourself more often than this, but I would strongly recommend no more than twice per week as you will only develop an obsession about your body weight. Focusing on every little change in your weight from meal to meal and from day to day is not what you should be doing as body weight can fluctuate by as much as 1 to 2 kilograms in any given day.

These day-to-day fluctuations are normal and expected. The meal-to-meal and day-to-day fluctuations that you witness in your body weight are due to hydration or the amount of water in your body, and not a true change in fat mass.

Weigh yourself on the same scales, at a similar time, and with the same clothing, or naked, each week. For consistency, first thing before breakfast is a good time. It is important to use the same set of scales as there can be a huge discrepancy between different scales, and cheap ones that are not calibrated will only return inaccurate and unreliable measurements. Choose scales with a large electronic display that makes it easy to read the weight, and be sure to change the batteries regularly. A body weight recording is the only thing you need. The majority of scales now provide all sorts of data, including body fat analysis, but they are largely misleading and inaccurate unless they are specific bioelectrical impedance analysis-type scales, and these are very expensive!

When observing your body weight the key is to analyse the trend of your weight over time. Remember, the weight will come off naturally if you can focus on putting aspects of the IWL plan into practice, and you have already calculated your realistic goal weight loss and know the amount you are allowed to lose each month. Record your weight on some form of tracker with every weigh-in and monitor the trend over the month. If you are in the middle of a weight-loss period, the trend should be going down 1 to 2 kilograms over the month, and if it is a weight-maintenance month it should be stable across the month in order to reset your body weight. You will never have a perfect weight trajectory – it is just the trend you are looking for.

Tracking your body weight will achieve the simple task of allowing you to get to know how your body works and responds to different stimuli. Later chapters teach you how to adjust your lifestyle in accordance with what your weight trajectory is doing. An example of a recording chart for both a weight-loss period and a weight-maintenance period is as follows:

(A)   Body weight tracker for weight-loss month

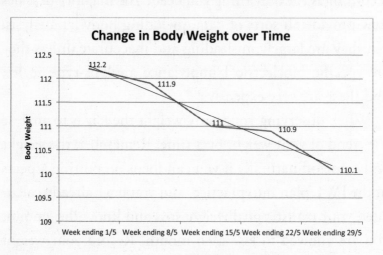

Note the trend is going down over the course of the month (approximate 2 kg weight loss from starting point – day 0 – of 112.2 kg). It is important to ensure you are not losing more than 0.5 kg per week. If you see it going down by more than 0.5 kg per week you need to take your foot off the accelerator and adjust your food or activity level, as outlined in Chapter 12. The black line is the linear trend, which is what you want to observe over time. No weight-loss trajectory is ever perfect. Don't panic if the weight loss is varying from week to week – this is normal. If you see the trend going down over the month, then you are perfectly on track!

(B) Body weight tracker for weight-maintenance month

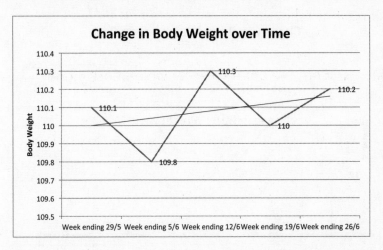

Note the trend evens out over the course of the month to maintain the 2 kg weight loss from the previous month. This is extremely important as continued weight loss will result in failure. The black line is the linear trend. In this graph, the variations in body weight are considered weight maintenance. Your weight should stay within 1 kg over the entire month.

(C) Body weight tracker for weight-maintenance month

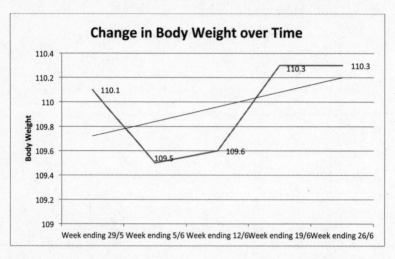

Note that in this instance there is a trend towards weight loss over the first two weeks (from 110.1 kg at the end of a weight-loss period in Figure A to 109.5 kg on week ending 5/6 and 109.6 kg on week ending 12/6). Because this is supposed to be a weight-maintenance period, the person has corrected this by allowing for a higher energy intake to ensure their body weight corrects back to the starting point of the weight-maintenance month (which was 110.1 kg – see Figure A). This will be further elaborated in Chapter 12. A weight trajectory from 110.1 to 110.3 kg over the month is considered weight maintenance and definitely not weight gain.

(D) Body weight tracker for 12-month period

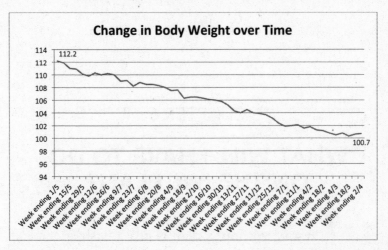

Note that in this 12-month chart the weight is decreasing by approximately 2 kg each month and then maintained for the following month, equating to approximately a 12 kg weight loss over an entire year. Body weight is 112.2 kg at baseline and 100.7 kg after approximately 12 months. You can see that some months have resulted in very little weight loss and others a little more. It will never be a perfect weight trajectory.

CHAPTER 6

WHAT WILL I HAVE TO DO ON THE IWL PLAN?

'A goal without a plan is just a wish'
– *Antoine de Saint-Exupry*

We know that weight loss is not just about what food we eat or how much exercise we do. Obesity and weight gain are multifactorial and complex problems, and challenging to address. It's also about how we structure and organise our day-to-day life, how we prevent emotional and comfort eating, and simple but important things like how much sleep we get. The IWL plan is about how to change your life for the better so that you start to prioritise your health and put into place a new approach that is sustainable for the rest of your life.

Meal plans and calorie counting

Many readers have asked me whether you need to follow a set meal plan and count calories on the Interval Weight Loss plan, so I'm sure what I'm about to say is music to their ears! No, absolutely not! It doesn't require you to do either. After all, no one wants to sit down and weigh out 60 grams of chicken or measure out 80 grams of rice, or look for activated almonds in the shops. (By the way, despite what you have been told there is no difference between the nutritional value of activated almonds and regular almonds. Nor is there a difference in the nutritional value of certain sugars such as muscovado, rapadura and demerara sugar, compared to regular white or brown sugar.)

The IWL plan is a simplistic, realistic and fun lifestyle that will see you develop a new passion for food and nutrition. You need to move away from the mentality of relying on set meal plans and counting calories. Weight loss is not as simple as calories in versus calories out. The body is far too complex for that. And who has time to weigh the ingredients for each meal?! Even if you did, it would make no difference. It's utter nonsense. For years we've been told to count calories, to only eat certain foods for breakfast, to avoid carbs at night, and so on. This only compounds the issue. We shouldn't be restricting but rather increasing our food intake from wholesome, nutritious foods.

I believe we also need to eat the majority of our food at the start of the day and less at the end. At the moment we seem to have it all wrong, with the majority of the population skipping breakfast only to see a huge spike in their hunger towards the end of the day. Consequently we overeat later in the day, particularly the evening meal.

By focusing on the foods that are outlined later in the book you will see a reduction in the amount of calories you are consuming without even focusing on it.

Ingrained mentalities

One of the most important things to understand is that the IWL plan is not something that you just 'have a go at' and see how you do. With that sort of attitude you will always fail. In fact, with that attitude you were doomed to fail before you began.

This has never been clearer to me than when I first published *Interval Weight Loss*. I made some TV appearances to promote the book which resulted in Channel 10 asking me to come back on their show and run a regular weight-loss segment. The result was the 'Studio 10 Interval Weight Loss Challenge', which began with a call-out to viewers to participate in a 12-month program under my guidance. I wanted to show that the IWL plan can be performed regardless of your day-to-day activities and by all.

Hundreds of people sent in their applications, but when I asked them to commit to a long-term plan they'd say, 'I just thought I could give it a go, see how it goes, and then you could film me if I was doing well.' This was exactly the type of patient I had seen in my clinics. They had given up before they even started – but once I changed their attitude to one of focus and persistence, these people succeeded, too.

Decluttering

One way to help yourself become focused is by decluttering. 'But hang on, isn't this a weight-loss book?' I hear you cry. 'Why do you want me to declutter?' Bear with me. One of the key parts of the IWL plan is leading a streamlined yet well-organised life – something keenly advocated by minimalists.

There are now so many great books written on the topic of minimalism and the art of decluttering that I don't intend to add to this section of the bookshop. But I will say that you will find it much harder to succeed if you continue to carry that excess baggage around with you and fail to let it go. What I am referring to here, specifically, is all those clothes you have been holding on to for many years in the hope that you will one day fit into them when you lose weight. One of the first things on your 'to do' list needs to be 'go through wardrobe'. Every item that you haven't worn for six months must go into the clothing bin, to someone in need. There are no 'what ifs' in this situation. Get rid of it and reward yourself with a trip to the shops when you reach your new 'set point' in months to come.

Holding on to all these things in life will not allow you to move on and break through into your new self.

It is important to let go of your old life, your old notions of the size you should be, your notions of a fashion ideal that never suited your body shape in the first place and anything that is a reminder of the old you. This will allow you to break through the wall and into your inner silhouette – the weight your body wants to be.

If you haven't used it or worn it in six months (or it has been through a season unused) either put it in the rubbish, or if still in good condition give it to someone in need. Use this checklist as a guide to help you achieve a life with less possessions and more happiness.

1. Make a list of all rooms, cupboards and drawers that need clearing out, including the garage or storage rooms if you have them.

2. Add one thing at a time to your 'to do' list – this will allow you to clear out the house section by section. Remember, this is a long game and not something that is achieved overnight.

3. Remove the TV and computer from your bedroom. This is a place for rest and should not in any way be associated with technological distraction. Research has repeatedly shown that the blue light emission will disturb your circadian rhythm and, consequently, your sleep.

4. If you have a piece of cardio equipment (such as a stationary bike), put it in front of the TV. This

is a gentle reminder to keep your sitting time to a minimum and will force you to either embrace it or get rid of it.

5. Last but not least, remove anything that's been abandoned on a flat surface. If it doesn't have a home it either needs to go or it needs to find a home. Your house doesn't need to look like it's out of a magazine, but it does need to look organised and neat.

The great thing about decluttering is that it keeps you engaged in constructive activities. While you are doing it, you are succeeding on the IWL plan because it will prevent you from sitting in front of the TV and involved in activities you are not even aware you're doing, like mindless eating.

The evening is the most challenging time for some of us, and by working through your 'to do' list after dinner or participating in a hobby (for example, building something with the kids or reading) you will be preoccupied and less likely to reach for those comfort foods.

Focus is not the same as an all-or-nothing approach

When you read this book and get your head around the concept of the IWL plan and its long-term focus, it must be a method that feels easy to incorporate into your life.

It's not an all-or-nothing approach that you see so often when someone starts a diet on a Monday after a weekend of bingeing.

There are no exclusions and no forced inclusions with the IWL plan because you only end up craving a particular food you have omitted, hating the new exercise you have started, or abandoning the hobby you have taken up. If the IWL plan starts to feel a little too much, I suspect you are still being over-zealous. The transition to nutritious and wholesome foods recommended in the IWL plan may take some getting used to, but you will get used to it, and you will feel better for it. Trust me!

CHAPTER 7

STRUCTURED PLANS AND HOW TO IMPLEMENT IWL

'There is nothing permanent except change'
– *Heraclitus*

On six out of seven days a week you need to follow a structured plan that consists of food prepared at home and the inclusion of regular activity. 'Structured' is not a euphemism for 'difficult' though. As I've just explained, planning ahead shouldn't feel arduous and it shouldn't feel like a chore.

The weight-loss months will require you to eat at home more diligently and to include more physical activity, and the weight-maintenance months will allow you to relax a little with your food intake and to reduce your physical activity to the minimum daily requirement (explained in later chapters). You need to plan each day and use action plans and 'to do' lists, but these will soon become second nature to you.

As kids we were told what to do, which meant we had discipline and routine imposed on us. As adults we need to tell ourselves what to do to keep us on track. Over the next few pages I will share some weekly structured IWL plans to give you a clear idea of how you might organise your week and what you can do to ensure you lose or maintain weight during each respective month.

You can and should make your own weekly IWL plan that fits your schedule, your priorities, your exercise preferences and your dietary requirements. For instance, the IWL plan of a vegetarian couple who both work full-time will be very different to that of a single, retired bowls enthusiast. The beauty of the IWL plan is that it is customisable to your personal needs. For the weight-loss months, base it on the following fundamental principles:

1. Five meals per day – biggest meal when you get up and smallest meal at the end of the day.

2. Home-cooked meals on six days per week – use leftovers each night for lunch the next day to make it simple and save yourself time and money.

3. One treat food per week (for example, an ice-cream) and one dining-out meal (for example, pizza).

4. 30 minutes of exercise six days per week, of varying intensity and different types of activity.

5. Sleep 6–8 hours per night.

6. TV-free days on three days per week.

7. No more than two hours TV per day on the other four days.

You'll see that point six mentions TV-free days, which I realise might be challenging at first. In practical terms, if you have a TV addiction, this means choosing your favourite shows and slowly reducing the amount of screen time you have by weaning yourself off it and working towards three TV-free days per week.

For the weight-maintenance months base it on the following fundamental principles:

1. Five meals per day – the biggest meal at the start and the smallest meal at the end of the day (note that there is no difference in portion size to the weight-loss month).

2. Home-cooked meals on five days per week – use leftovers each night for lunch the next day to make this simple.

3. Two treat foods and two dining-out meals per week if you live close to restaurants and can afford it. This can be substituted by cooking a treat meal at home.

4. 30 minutes of exercise on five days per week of low to moderate intensity without a need to vary the type of activity each day.

5. Sleep 6–8 hours per night.

6. TV-free days on two days per week.

7. No more than two hours of TV per day on the other five days.

EXAMPLE WEEK OF A WEIGHT-LOSS MONTH

Some people use their weekends to turbocharge their weight-loss goals, and some prefer to relax and focus during the week. This plan is just a suggestion – you have to work out what suits you.

The first thing to organise is your exercise routine. Guidelines for general health say you should do at least five 30-minute exercise sessions per week (this can be brisk walking). You need to work out how that fits into your lifestyle and you need to mix up the duration, type of exercise, and intensity of exercise to ensure you achieve your weight-loss goal during the weight-loss months.

With the following plan, each day will also be accompanied by a large morning tea and small afternoon tea to ensure you have five meals per day. These meals can be selected from the *Reference Guide* provided at the back of the book – a guide that should be copied and stuck on your fridge at home and put in a place visible to you at work.

Lastly, this weekly plan includes reference to some of the recipes at the back of this book. You don't have to stick to these recipes – they're simply there to emphasise the type of ingredients you should use as the foundations for all recipes, and to show you how easy it can be to cook. The recipes are designed specifically to be simple and are aimed at busy people who don't have time to find lots of obscure ingredients. Your time is too valuable to spend it hunting for cacao extract at the health food store!

Sunday

In our house, Sunday is the day we grocery shop and get organised for the week (note that there is a detailed grocery list that you can use as the basis of your shopping in Chapter 8). You could use the shopping outing as an opportune time for activity by walking or riding to the shops so that carrying your groceries becomes part of your exercise regime.

Sunday might also be a time to run around the playground with your kids or to take some time for yourself at the gym or the yoga studio. For us, it's also a day of the week where we tend to the vegetable garden. Sometimes we harvest a lot of this produce to make something we can freeze (such as the Pesto-infused Potato, Zucchini and

Leek Soup on page 171) and then have for lunch or dinner on a couple of days during the week. We also make a batch of muesli (page 159) for breakfast during the week. The following is a sample Sunday:

Brekkie – Miso Scrambled Eggs with Vegetables (page 160), and skim milk coffee.

Morning tea – See *Reference Guide* – Foods you can eat when hungry (page 263).

Lunch – Chicken or tuna and salad wholegrain sandwich.

Afternoon tea – See *Reference Guide* – Foods you can eat when hungry (page 263).

Dinner – Sally's Vegetable Risotto (page 225). *Hot tip: make double the serving and enjoy for lunch on Monday.*

After dinner – Watch some TV while riding the stationary bike. It doesn't have to be intense, just lightly turn the legs over. It will keep your mind off food. You need to shift your mindset to avoid the dependence on food when relaxing (comfort eating) or when in front of technology. Whenever you think you're hungry have a glass of water or a cup of herbal tea first to make sure that it is 'true' hunger and not a sign of comfort eating.

Bed – 10 pm for 8 hours sleep. Even if you find yourself struggling to go to sleep because you have been going to bed late for decades, this is a mindset you need to shift – try reading or listening to relaxation music, practise meditation, or listen to a podcast.

Monday

Start your week off the right way by getting up 30 minutes earlier than normal and going for a walk. Ensure you track your incidental activity every day and aim for 10,000 steps at a minimum.

Brekkie – Avocado on wholegrain toast with skim milk coffee.

Morning tea – See *Reference Guide* – Foods you can eat when hungry (page 263).

Lunch – Leftover risotto from the night before.

Afternoon tea – See *Reference Guide* – Foods you can eat when hungry (page 263).

Dinner – Delicious Crispy-skin Salmon with Greens (page 201). This meal may not keep well for leftovers the next day so cook enough just for the evening meal.

After dinner – Work on something on your 'to do' list. It might be 'Clean out kitchen cupboards' or 'Go through clothes for charity'. It doesn't matter which item you choose on your 'to do' list, all that matters is that it keeps you busy and stops you thinking about food. 'To do' lists also keep you organised and constructive. Importantly, they help you develop confidence in yourself and bring a positive attitude and successful routine into your life. You have to learn to praise yourself for the simple things in life and it is very satisfying to have a physical list that you actively cross things off as you complete them. The 'to do' list can be written on paper or in your phone, and can include anything that needs to be done. It will be an evolving list that sometimes seems bigger than Ben Hur and at other times makes you feel as though you are on top of the world. It doesn't matter what is on your list, it just matters that there is a list.

Bed – 10 pm for 8 hours sleep.

Tuesday

Brekkie – Avocado on wholegrain toast with skim milk coffee.

Morning tea – See *Reference Guide* – Foods you can eat when hungry (page 263).

Lunch – Meal prepared from Sunday that was in the freezer (such as the soup).

Afternoon tea – See *Reference Guide* – Foods you can eat when hungry (page 263).

After work – Hit the gym, or if that's not for you try an at-home YouTube workout for 30 minutes. If you don't have any equipment, do a body-weight session or use tins of chickpeas as your weights. The most important thing here is that you do a session or gym routine that you have never done before. I recommend varying your exercise and incorporating a range of activities every day of the week. On the days you are pushed for time, aim for high-intensity, short-duration activities (like a gym workout), and on days when time is on your side, aim for a low-intensity, long-duration activity (like swimming laps).

Dinner – Vegetable pizzas.
Don't be confused by the inclusion of pizza. Pizza, when it's made at home and covered in veggies, is not only *not* bad, it's good for you! Use a wholemeal-based pita bread or try making your own dough; load it up with veggies and it will be sure to fill you up. Just go easy on the cheese! It only needs a very light sprinkle to bind the ingredients together.

After dinner – Go for a gentle evening stroll to get you out of the house.

Bed – 10 pm for 8 hours sleep.

Wednesday

Brekkie – Porridge with frozen berries and skim milk.

Morning tea – See *Reference Guide* – Foods you can eat when hungry (page 263).

Lunch – Leftover vegetable pizza from the night before.

Afternoon tea – See *Reference Guide* – Foods you can eat when hungry (page 263).

Dinner – Cauliflower Rice, Chicken and Cashew Salad (page 183).

After dinner – Work on your 'to do' list. If you have kids, get them involved or if they have homework, help them with it.

Bed – 10 pm for 8 hours sleep.
Fight the 'hump day' mentality. Don't let yourself fall into the trap of wishing your life away and racing towards the weekend. Make the most of every day and make each day count.

Do something that you love. It could be a team sport, cycling with your kids, or having friends over for a healthy meal – why limit it to the weekend? In our house, we're fans of stand-up paddle-boarding and running laps around ovals (yes, really!) but we don't do the same session each time. We always mix it up.

Thursday

Keep up the good work! You've been exercising all week, why stop now? Get up early and mix up your commute. Ride your bike, get off a stop early, walk instead of driving. Just make sure you keep doing something different. Your body will only change if you provide it with a different stress.

Brekkie – Eggs (cooked to your liking) with pan-fried green veggies.

Who says veggies aren't a breakfast food?! Veggies should be fitted in whenever you can.

Morning tea – See *Reference Guide* – Foods you can eat when hungry (page 263).

Lunch – Leftover salad from the night before.

Afternoon tea – See *Reference Guide* – Foods you can eat when hungry (page 263).

Dinner – Crunchy Chickpea and Miso Black Rice Bowl (page 203).

After dinner – Play a board game, read a book, or dedicate some time to one of your hobbies.

Bed – 10 pm for 8 hours sleep.

Friday

Brekkie – Oven-baked Nutty Muesli (page 159) with frozen berries, honey and skim milk.

Morning tea – See *Reference Guide* – Foods you can eat when hungry (page 263).

Lunch – Leftover rice bowl from the night before.

Afternoon tea – See *Reference Guide* – Foods you can eat when hungry (page 263).

Dinner – Go out! It's Friday! Why not?
I don't advocate total deprivation on the IWL plan. It's all about treating yourself and maintaining a sustainable new

lifestyle. But make sure it's worth it. If it's pizza you love, don't waste a takeaway on average pizza, get the best pizza you can find! If you minimise the frequency of dining out to once a week during the weight-loss month you can have any favourite food.

Saturday

Brekkie – Baked Beans (page 163) on wholegrain toast.

Morning tea – See *Reference Guide* – Foods you can eat when hungry (page 263).

Lunch – Healthy Nachos (page 205)

Afternoon tea – See *Reference Guide* – Foods you can eat when hungry (page 263).

Dinner – Barbecue with salad. Alternatively why not have a Saturday picnic? Stroll from your house to a park, lake or beach nearby and reap the benefits of being in nature. Not only will you get your steps up walking there, it's a wonderful way to relax.

Treat – Gelato at your local Italian shop (note this is the one treat for the week).

EXAMPLE WEEK OF A WEIGHT-MAINTENANCE MONTH

This is a sample week from a weight-maintenance month of the IWL plan. As per the weekly plan provided for the weight-loss month, it's just a guide. You have to work out what works for you.

Exercise: Minimum 30 minutes of structured activity on five of the seven days. Allow yourself a little more flexibility as this month is simply about keeping up the exercise without having to think about what you need to do to vary it.

Food: Five meals per day. Morning and afternoon tea can be selected from the *Reference Guide* provided at the back of the book – a guide that should be written down onto paper and stuck on your fridge at home and placed somewhere visible at work. The meal structure stays the same as the weight-loss months but you can allow yourself more treats or dining-out meals.

Sunday

Brekkie – Walk to the bakery and pick up your favourite bread. If it's too far, try riding your bike there. Who says we have to drive everywhere? Enjoy a slice of bread with an omelette and a homemade coffee while having a relaxing morning reading the paper or your book.

Morning tea – See *Reference Guide* – Foods you can eat when hungry (page 263).

Lunch – Kimchi Stir-fry (page 209).

Afternoon tea – See *Reference Guide* – Foods you can eat when hungry (page 263).

Dinner – Delicious Lamb Shanks (page 211). This dish takes a while to cook so we usually make it on a Sunday. Shanks aren't the most practical food for lunch the next day at work, so I usually bring something from the freezer.

After dinner – Get away from the TV and work on one of your hobbies or tasks that needs completing. Sunday evening is a great time to read or do the paperwork that seems to be accumulating. It's also a great time to cook one of your favourite meals to freeze and use for lunches throughout the week. It might even be one of your treat days – remember, you can have two dining-out meals in the weight-maintenance month. Enjoy your favourite treat at the movies, and if it's feasible try riding your bike there rather than driving.

Bed – 10 pm for 8 hours sleep.

Monday

This work week you don't need to focus on exercise intensity or variety. And it's certainly not a time to increase the amount of exercise you are doing. The weight-maintenance months are not about sweat and pain. The focus is simply on continuing to move and ingraining those positive behaviours. Your weight won't go up if you keep up the movement. Aim to achieve your 10,000 steps per day but you can do it without having to sweat.

Brekkie – Fruit with low-fat Greek yoghurt, and skim milk coffee.

Morning tea – See *Reference Guide* – Foods you can eat when hungry (page 263).

Lunch – Meal from the freezer, such as soup.

Afternoon tea – See *Reference Guide* – Foods you can eat when hungry (page 263).

Dinner – Poke bowl (see page 187).

After dinner – Go for an evening stroll or work on your hobby.

Bed – 10 pm for 8 hours sleep.

Tuesday

Brekkie – Hummus on wholegrain toast with skim milk coffee.
Get in some early morning activity and do it while enjoying the sunrise. There is no better time of day than daybreak. You will feel energetic and vitalised before heading into work for the day.

Morning tea – See *Reference Guide* – Foods you can eat when hungry (page 263).

Lunch – Leftover poke bowl from the evening before.

Afternoon tea – See *Reference Guide* – Foods you can eat when hungry (page 263).

Dinner – Family-favourite Spaghetti Bolognese (page 199) with side salad. Pasta is a wonderful meal to make in large batches, but remember that half of the meal should be the accompanying salad.

After dinner – Enjoy some TV but do watch while riding the stationary bike. If you don't have a bike, do some sit-ups, or even sit down to a cup of herbal tea to distract yourself from eating.

Bed – 10 pm for 8 hours sleep.

Wednesday

Brekkie – Wholegrain toast with jam, and serving of yoghurt and fruit.

Morning tea – See *Reference Guide* – Foods you can eat when hungry (page 263).

Lunch – Leftover Spaghetti Bolognese from the night before.

Afternoon tea – See *Reference Guide* – Foods you can eat when hungry (page 263).

Dinner – Go out! Who says you have to wait till the weekend? Break up your week and dine out or order your favourite takeaway.

After dinner – Relax and unwind. Enjoy what's left of the day.

Bed – 11 pm for 7 hours sleep.

It's not always realistic to go to bed at the same time each night, especially if you have to go to a function one evening. The goal needs to be 6–8 hours per night. It is much better to wake up naturally than to the sound of an alarm.

Thursday

Brekkie – Wholegrain toast with avocado and smoked salmon.

Morning tea – See *Reference Guide* – Foods you can eat when hungry (page 263).

Lunch – Bring in a sandwich from home. Any sandwich is fine but make it with wholegrain bread and include salad.

Afternoon tea – See *Reference Guide* – Foods you can eat when hungry (page 263).

Dinner – Barbecue with sweet potato and zucchini chips. For the chips, simply chop up some sweet potato and zucchini into thin strips, spray with a little olive oil and throw them on the barbecue.

After dinner – Action something on your 'to do' list. If you have kids, get them involved. There is nothing more rewarding than seeing your own work come to fruition.

What things have you been meaning to do for ages but haven't completed yet? Put them on your 'to do' list and start to work through them.

Bed – 10 pm for 8 hours sleep.

Friday

Brekkie – Oats with honey and skim milk.
If practical, trial a different means of getting to work to focus on your incidental activity. Sometimes it's just as beneficial to incorporate movement into your day without having to go to a specific place to exercise. You could get off a stop early and walk part of the way to work, or even run if you're feeling particularly energetic.

Morning tea – See *Reference Guide* – Foods you can eat when hungry (page 263).

Lunch – Leftovers from the barbecue the night before.

Afternoon tea – See *Reference Guide* – Foods you can eat when hungry (page 263).

Dinner – Enjoy your second dining-out meal of the week! Follow this with your favourite treat.

This month is all about allowing yourself a little more leniency. The IWL plan is certainly not about total deprivation just because the diets you've tortured yourself with in the past have encouraged it. Remember, you might be able to abstain in the short term but you won't be able to stick to this approach in the long run.

Saturday

Brekkie – Fried eggs on wholegrain toast with avocado and smoked salmon.

Morning tea – See *Reference Guide* – Foods you can eat when hungry (page 263).

Lunch – Make some pizzas with your favourite toppings. Load them up with veggies and make them on wholemeal pita bases with a light sprinkle of cheese on each one.

Afternoon tea – See *Reference Guide* – Foods you can eat when hungry (page 263).

Dinner – Beef, Carrot, Potato and Cabbage Stew (page 191).

Evening – Go for a stroll around the neighbourhood, or relax and enjoy some of your favourite TV series or a movie.

Keep the frequency of dining out to twice a week and your treats to twice per week during the weight-maintenance month. Assess your weight at the end of the first week of this month. Don't panic if your weight goes up, just ensure you make the necessary changes for the coming week. And if it goes down, ensure you put the right actions into place to make sure it doesn't keep going down the following month (more on this later).

CHAPTER 8

BUYING THE RIGHT FOOD

'Let food be thy medicine and medicine be thy food' – *Hippocrates*

Food is the life source we need in order to nourish the body and help it get back to its natural preferred weight – its *set point*. It is important to focus on eating an abundance of foods and, if anything, to eat more – as long as it's wholesome, nutritious food.

When you embrace healthy eating (see the list later in this chapter) you will lose the fear of food that you have had for so long and it will become something you enjoy and that fuels your life, rather than something that controls you. You'll lose the belief that the more you eat the fatter you will become (as so many of my patients have thought), and you will also see the number on the scales go down. Inadvertently, the increase in food and change in foods you are eating will result in a reduction in your calorie intake. Our body needs good, nutritious food, and lots of it, as it is easier to process and allows our body to flourish. If you restrict the amount you eat it will only result in your body's functioning slowing down and you won't get the weight-loss results you are after.

Eat for the body you want, not for the body you have

In many instances, my patients don't actually start to lose weight until they *increase* their food intake. It seems ridiculous, I know, but remember the body will slow down during times of restriction and speed up during times of nourishment. The other important thing to remember, as I've outlined earlier, is that the IWL plan doesn't require you to sit down and record meticulously every piece of food you put into your body. There's nothing to be gained from obsessively recording calories in an app. This is because all calories are different. One classic example is nuts. We don't absorb all the calories when we eat nuts – they increase our resting energy expenditure, and they fill us up for long periods of time. So even though they are a source of fat, albeit a good source, their calorie content is not an accurate reflection of what your body is absorbing.

The good news is that you can take the painful task of calorie counting out of your weight-loss plan. And the other thing you don't need to do is weigh out foods or painstakingly wander the supermarket aisles for hours looking for so-called 'clean' ingredients that are no different in nutritional value but two to three times the price of their counterparts. The IWL plan brings back the pleasure to food that so many lose when they obsessively diet, meaning people find it an easy and sustainable approach to changing their lifestyle.

The basis of your daily food intake should include the following foods:

1. Fruit and vegetables (all are suitable but enjoy a variety). Yes, that's right, there are NO bad fruits or vegetables. Despite what you've been told, bananas and potatoes are fine to eat and are in fact key weapons in your weight-loss arsenal.

2. Plenty (two to three serves per day) of skim or low-fat dairy (milk and yoghurt). Cheese, when eaten by itself, should be kept to only once per week. If opting for dairy alternatives, choose soy products that specify on the label 'calcium-fortified' or 'calcium-enriched'.

3. A handful of nuts and seeds (as a guide 30–60 g, but double this is fine). If buying in bulk, portion them out to avoid mindless eating.

4. Wholegrain carbohydrate, preferably with three meals per day. Wholegrains, or foods made with them,

contain all components of the original grain seed (i.e. the bran, germ and endosperm). All of these must be present to qualify as a wholegrain. For example, wholegrain bread, wholegrain pasta, brown rice, barley, buckwheat, steel-cut oats, quinoa. Couscous and white rice are not wholegrains so should not be as prevalent in the diet as their wholegrain cousins.

5. Plenty of fish (any type is fine) and seafood with at least three meals per week.

6. Inclusion of protein – lean or 'heart smart' cuts of meat (trim all visible forms of fat off the meat), or legumes (all types), or eggs with each of the three main meals per day. Focusing on including more legumes and eggs instead of meat during the weight-loss months is particularly important. You don't need meat with every meal and legumes are a nutritionally sound alternative to help you achieve your goals on the weight-loss months.

7. Treats no more than once per week (e.g. ice-cream, chocolate, biscuits). These must be portion-controlled, so buy chocolates or ice-creams in individual packaging, or divvy biscuits into separate containers to avoid eating the whole packet or tub.

8. Fast food or dining out no more than once per week.

9. A glass of water before every meal and at times when you think you are hungry.

Patients of mine have often found it helpful to write this list of foods down and keep it on their fridge so that it's visible every time they visit the kitchen. Note that at the back of the book there is also a guide to foods you should eat when you're hungry.

Grocery shopping

Grocery shopping is not easy. Supermarkets are designed to guide us around the perimeter of the store and to make short trips up and down the aisles. Unsurprisingly, therefore, products located at the end of the aisles and at checkout counters account for nearly half of all sales. They are stacked with soft drinks, sweets, chips and bakery goods.

To limit your exposure to these foods, your grocery shopping should be done once a week. If you really don't trust yourself in the supermarket you should consider ordering everything online and having it delivered. It is much better to do that than succumb to those impulse buys and poor food choices when at the supermarket. In addition, the extra time you've saved from that risky shopping expedition can be devoted to some structured physical activity or one of your hobbies. The weekly food shop will not change much from week to week, which makes ordering online even easier as your foods will be saved from the previous week's purchase.

If you're going to hit the shops, it's important to take a list with you so you don't forget anything and have to go back to the supermarket mid-week. Not only is it a good way to make smart food choices, it can save you money. It's also sensible to break up the shopping so that you conquer it in sections. Get your fruit and veg from your local fruit shop, your meat from your local butcher, and your staples from one of the supermarket chains. The amount of money you can save by shopping at one of the discount wholesaler chains is incredible. Sure, you might not get the same variety in product choice but it makes the shopping experience a whole lot easier when you can't dither between six different types of pesto.

It is important to only go shopping *after* eating a meal (preferably after breakfast, which is the biggest and most important meal of the day). This will prevent those impulse buys that we are inclined to make when we visit the supermarket hungry. Going to the supermarket on an empty stomach results in disaster as we find ourselves reaching for anything we can get our hands on, namely those convenient, energy-dense, nutrient-poor foods coming out of a packet. Everyone's found themselves at the checkout munching on chips before you've even bought them, right?

The majority of the shopping can be done on the fringe or outside section of the supermarket (though, as

I've said, be wary of the ends of aisles), which is where all the fresh produce is located. There are several aisles that can be skipped altogether, which are loaded with foods coming out of a packet and offer very little nutrition. Skip the chips and the confectionary when you're at the supermarket, so that you won't be tempted by them inside the house. It's much easier than being haunted by a block of chocolate, night after night.

As you know, there are *no* foods that are excluded in the IWL plan, but there are foods that should be kept to a minimum of once per week in the weight-loss months. The following foods need to be kept in the 'treat' basket. This doesn't mean you can have all these food items, though, it means you need to select your favourite! The great news is you can have them more often during the weight-maintenance months.

Treats:

- Chips
- Biscuits
- Snack bars, energy bars, or muesli bars
- Lollies
- Chocolate
- Dried fruit
- White bread
- Savouries and pastries
- Ice-cream.

Basically anything processed should be thought of as a treat food. Clever marketing and misleading food packaging make things confusing, so be aware that just because something is labelled 'health food', 'gluten-free', 'dairy-free', 'wheat-free' or 'vegan' doesn't mean it is better for you. It will still be loaded with added sugar and fat and needs to be thought of as a treat.

The foods on this list are very low in nutrition (or have no nutrition) and/or are packed full of calories. Chocolate is more nutritious when it has more than 70 per cent cocoa content, but is still most certainly a treat as it's packed full of calories. Most concerning is that it's one of those foods we reach for very commonly after dinner when we sit down to relax.

Then there is cheese! This needs to be kept to once per week, or on two occasions if part of a meal (as with the pizzas in the suggested IWL plans in Chapter 7), but can be enjoyed in addition to the treats listed above. Cheese is often one of those foods that we cut up and snack on as we prepare the evening meal, only to devour an entire day's calorie intake in a one-hour sitting. It's also something we tend to eat a lot of without noticing. For example, when you go to a dinner party or a get-together with friends in Australia it's often served before the meal (this isn't common in other countries, where cheese is served after the meal), and you tend to graze on it as you chat. You need to go easy at these times so it's best to ensure you don't arrive at the dinner party hungry.

By limiting your cheese intake, you will look to other food options before dinner which contain the same nutrition but half (or possibly even more than half) the calories. Milk and yoghurt are two such examples when you're at home. But nuts are another great snack alternative, particularly if you are required to shell them before eating as it slows down your consumption. You could also get stuck into some homemade hummus (see page 237) or chopped up vegetables such as carrot and cucumber.

Curbing the sugar craving

It's one thing for me to tell you to only have treats once per week but it's another to put this into action. As discussed earlier, since the industrial revolution we have sought pleasure from fast food and processed foods that are packed with sugar, salt and fat, triggering addictive-like eating behaviours. Eating sugar lights up the brain's dopamine receptors making us feel good at the time. We then race around not long after looking for another hit – often the rest of the packet of chocolate. Anything and everything that is processed is addictive and it tastes good. Before the industrial revolution we got our sugar hit from nature's naturally occurring sources of sugar: fruit.

Reflect back to the first chapter. It takes time to change behaviour – 66 days, in fact! The dieting mentality of simply cutting out foods we love and are addicted to simply does not work. We always end up going back for more. There is a reason we are addicted to them and, just like any other addiction, you will need to gradually wean yourself off these foods.

Try these tips for curbing your desire for fast food and processed foods:

1. If you are currently eating a bakery treat every day (it might be a cupcake, muffin or doughnut) or getting takeaway every day, reduce the frequency of these foods gradually. Slowly work towards an intake of one treat per week on the weight-loss months of the IWL plan and to two per week on the weight-maintenance months. This will also allow you to gradually accept the concept of more home cooking and food preparation at home. It may take longer to achieve your goal with this weaning process but it's an effective approach.

2. Find some fruits that you love and surround yourself with them. Every time you feel that urge to eat something sugary coming on, eat some fruit instead. You will get the same high you usually get, as naturally occurring sugars found in fruit also light up our brain's dopamine receptors. Better still, the cravings will eventually fade. Be prepared, though, to ride out that 66-day barrier to break down the wall. It's worth it.

3. Buy single serve packages of chocolate, ice-cream, biscuits, chips or whatever your favourite treats might

be. This enforces the portion size and reduces the risk of you devouring the entire packet.

4. Keep the treats out of sight so you do not see them every time you open the fridge or cupboard. Keep healthy foods visible and at eye level at all times.

5. Every time you get a sugar craving, try taking just a taste. By allowing yourself a few bites you get maximum enjoyment for minimal damage. Research has proven this – the first bite of any treat food yields the most pleasure!

6. Cut down on impulse eating by delaying pleasure. For example, tell yourself you can have the McDonald's, Pizza Hut, chocolate bar or ice-cream after you complete that task on your 'to do' list. You make it harder to access the treat but are not saying no. Patients of mine often find they replace their sugar craving with the pleasure of completing a task. They forget all about food because they are so happy they have finished a job and want to continue while they're on a roll.

7. Record your expenditure. A simple task that involves recording all your food intake can often prompt you to eat out less often and to buy fewer treats and takeaway. Buying food on the go or convenience foods all the time can be very expensive. You can usually get four home-cooked meals for the price of

one dining-out meal, which will have a huge effect on your bank balance over time and also make you more aware of your food choices.

Shopping list

To avoid being overwhelmed on your first grocery shop, the following list can be used, and can form the basis of your grocery shopping. This can be tailored to some of your preferences, or food eating practices such as vegetarianism.

If you're really time-poor and are in the financial position to do so, you could consider the meal-delivery services that are now on offer (they will send you different ingredients and recipes to cook for the week). They are certainly very popular at the moment and it means you don't have to think about what's for dinner. But the catch! People become bored of it, just as they do with all commercial programs and products, and end up going back to their old habits when the novelty has worn off.

Shopping for yourself is always going to be more satisfying, nutritionally balanced and generate less packaging. It should be the first preference. I suggest the following:

Breads: Wholegrain bread and wholegrain pita bread to use for wraps. Ensure the words 'whole wheat' or 'whole wheat flour' is the first ingredient on the label. Buy the bread that is darkest in appearance and full of grains.

Pasta: Wholegrain pasta ideally; however, any pasta is fine to buy as the focus of any pasta dish needs to be the meal balance. You should eat pasta with an accompanying salad so that half of your portion is the pasta and the other half the salad.

Cereals: Steel-cut oats, natural muesli and any wholegrain-based cereals such as Weet-Bix or All-Bran. When you are in the cereal aisle, avoid all the processed cereals with added sugar as they will leave you starving by 9 am.

Rice: Brown rice, basmati rice. Also consider alternative grains like quinoa or barley, but don't feel you have to include them if you don't like them, can't find them or can't afford them.

Meat: Chicken or turkey breasts, or other cuts without the skin; 'heart smart' mince, or lean cuts of beef. The cheaper cuts of meat from a cow tend to be the toughest, such as blade and porterhouse, and are best for slow-cooked dishes where the protein breaks down over time to give it its tenderness. This is fine and makes a difference only to your wallet and method of cooking.

Lamb is a great alternative to beef and packed full of flavour, but unless you can afford the premium cuts it is a much fattier meat, so limit things like lamb chops to once per week.

Keep all varieties of pork to a maximum of once per week as it often comes in a processed form such as bacon, and is a much fattier meat alternative to beef and chicken.

Lastly, keep processed meats like sliced meats, chorizo or salami to the 'treat' category as they are preserved with additives and salt to prolong their shelf life.

Tip: It is easy to pick out the leanest cuts of meat as they will have less marbling or white fatty tissue visible. The white part is the fat.

Seafood: All seafood is nutritious and you can include any type. Yes, even shellfish, such as prawns, are excellent food sources. Despite the myth about prawns, shellfish won't increase the cholesterol level in the blood – unless you're eating them covered in batter!

Oils: Canola oil or olive oil only, both bottled and spray. Any variety of olive oil is fine. Extra virgin is not refined and better for salads due to its more pungent flavour. Standard olive oil is better suited for cooking and baking. If you can't afford olive oil, choose canola oil. Coconut oil is not something you should be eating despite it being the centre of one of the best marketing scams of the 21st century, nor is rice bran oil or any of the trendy alternatives. Government nutrition guidelines specifically state to avoid coconut oil because of its detrimental effect on heart health. Keeping a bottle of sesame oil on hand is helpful for dishes where you need the occasional teaspoon of it.

Condiments: Low salt and low added sugar tomato sauce, wholegrain mustard, tomato paste, stock cubes or pre-made stock. Condiments such as mayonnaise, aioli and barbecue sauce should be kept to a minimum because of their dense calorie content and minimal nutritional value.

Canned food: Tomatoes, lentils, chickpeas, tuna, salmon, fruit in natural juice, low-salt vegetable soup. Jarred garlic and ginger (no added sugar or salt) are practical alternatives to fresh produce, but be aware that they are much less flavoursome and you can notice the difference in cooking.

Frozen food: Frozen vegetables, frozen fruit, reduced-fat frozen yoghurt. Frozen vegetables are snap-frozen as they are harvested, and therefore retain the same level of nutrients as fresh vegetables (ignore people who say that they aren't as good for you). They also allow people to enjoy raspberries and blueberries in the dead of winter and other veggies out of season, plus they're often cheaper than their fresh counterparts.

Dairy: Skim or low-fat milk and yoghurt, low-fat cottage cheese. Opt for plain yoghurt and add your own sweetness by using fruit or honey. If you can't tolerate dairy, calcium-fortified soy milk is an acceptable alternative, but be aware that it doesn't contain iodine (iodine deficiency is becoming more common across the globe and it is a nutrient essential for thyroxine production in the body – a hormone that controls your weight). Almond milk is often extremely sweetened, full of water and low in protein, so be wary of it.

Fresh produce: Eggs, avocado, fruits, vegetables.

Snacks and spreads: Nuts (a mix including almonds and walnuts – natural or dry-roasted), seeds (for example, pumpkin, sunflower and sesame seeds), wholegrain crackers, chocolate (preferably greater than 70 per cent cocoa content), peanut butter (100 per cent peanuts), or any other form of nut butter (for example, cashew butter, almond butter), fruit spread (no added sugar), Vegemite.

It's better not to use butter or margarine so stick to olive oil or avocado as your spread of choice.

Beverages: Tea, coffee, sparkling water. Coffee and tea are good for your health but try not to have more than two cups per day due to the stimulant effect of caffeine. Also be sure to avoid it after 4 pm as caffeine can disrupt your sleep or ability to fall asleep.

CHAPTER 9

USE CHOPSTICKS

*'It's when you eat jelly beans with chopsticks
that people begin to think you're crazy'
– Anthony T. Hincks*

Breakfast is the most important meal so ensure you are well prepared and focus on eating the majority of your food at the beginning of the day. You must then taper off the volume of food you eat so that lunch becomes the next biggest meal of the day with dinner as the smallest.

The evening can be one of the trickiest times when it comes to overeating. We get home tired at the end of the day, are ravenous and reach for anything we can get our hands on. The reason we are often hungry is that we've neglected to eat for the majority of the day, using lack of time and lack of hunger as excuses. You will always fail to be hungry at the start of the day and not feel the need for breakfast if you overeat every night, and you will never have time to sit down and eat properly if you devote everything to work and nothing to yourself. Food preparation is the key. If you take food with you as you leave home every day you are planning for success. And if you set alarms on your phone to prompt you to eat and enjoy the food away from technological distraction, you will not neglect to eat or end up looking for emergency food.

The other issue in the evening is that we associate food preparation or the end of the work day with winding down, and consequently snacking and drinking. Is this because it was a stressful day? Eating and drinking are certainly the last things we should do to de-stress and unwind. Why? Because they just serve as a quick fix and although it might feel good at the time it doesn't feel good the next morning when you wake up with a foggy head, the guilty feeling of poor food choices or overeating, or the hangover.

You will only be able to avoid the excessive hunger in the afternoon if you eat more at the start of the day and focus the majority of your food intake from breakfast to lunch. You should then have a small afternoon meal before you leave work for the day, or on your way home. This will prevent the common hunger pangs you experience every day when you get home from work and reach for a packet of chips.

If it has been a stressful day, don't jump straight into the cooking. Instead, if it's practical for you, burn out a quick 20-minute exercise session to get those endorphins pumping around the body and to alleviate stress. It doesn't matter what the exercise is, all that matters is that you address the stress before putting yourself in an environment where you are tempted to self-medicate with alcohol and junk food, or the high-calorie comfort foods. Cheese is usually high on the list!

Dinner is the most important meal from a social and cultural perspective and should be eaten away from technological distraction and preferably at the dinner table (just like every other meal throughout the day). It also needs to be served on a tiny plate or very small bowl and eaten with chopsticks. Yes, you read that correctly! Chopsticks!

If you have never learnt to use chopsticks, now is the time. It can be very frustrating and difficult at first but you will eventually get the hang of it. The more uncomfortable you are with them, the better, as it will force you to eat even slower. The whole point of incorporating chopsticks into the evening meal is to slow you down. Don't give up if you don't master the use of chopsticks straight away.

Slowing down your meal and serving up less food at the evening meal allows time for signals to be sent from your stomach to your brain to tell you you're full. We are hardwired to eat huge portions at dinner and don't give our bodies a chance to tell us we don't need any more food. The only way to give yourself the opportunity to listen to your body's cues is by forcing yourself to eat slower, and hence the use of the chopsticks.

What to do if you're still hungry

Give your brain time to gauge its fullness and listen to your appetite hormones. If you're still hungry after the first serve, wait five minutes before going back for a second. If you are still hungry after your second serve, you are either still eating too quickly (but this is unlikely unless you are a master of the chopsticks!), or you simply didn't focus the majority of your food intake in the morning. In the case of the latter you need to adjust how much food you are eating in the morning to give yourself a chance of eating less at dinner.

Where you are hungry because you have messed up your eating for the day – for example, meetings got in the way – don't panic. In this instance, it is important to have emergency foods around, like fruit, dairy products and nuts so that you don't go and binge on sweets or foods from the vending machine if you are still in the office.

Although you will be eating less at dinner, it is still the most important meal from a social and cultural perspective. For some it's a time where you can chat about your day, or perhaps write in a journal as you eat if you live alone. Conversation or writing notes in a journal will both slow down your eating.

There are recipes at the back of the book with suggested portions, but these are only a guide and it is better to cook more food so that you, your partner, or your kids can have leftovers the following day. As we don't have time to prepare all of our meals from scratch every day, utilising leftovers for lunch is a perfect way to stop you eating out, keeping you on track with your IWL plan.

CHAPTER 10

MIXING UP YOUR EXERCISE ROUTINE

'Quality is not an act, it is a habit' – *Aristotle*

The ability to walk on two legs is one of the earliest defining human traits, and evolved around six million years ago. Movement was needed to survive, but evolution has seen humans transition from a nomadic lifestyle, hunting for food with a body designed for walking long distances, to a sedentary lifestyle sitting in front of screens.

Very few of us are meeting the measly two-and-a-half hours of activity per week recommended to keep healthy. At just half an hour of moderate activity on five days of the week, it's something that two in three people aren't doing. Following the IWL plan, you will become the exception to the rule!

Even fewer people do the recommended two days per

week of muscle-strengthening exercises – something that is, even when executed in the convenience of your own home, associated with a 20 per cent lower chance of dying prematurely. One in 10 deaths worldwide are attributable to physical inactivity. We are simply not moving enough and it is a large part of the reason for the bulging waist-lines we see today.

Sarco-what?

To compound the issue even more, our muscle mass naturally declines at around 40 years and this decline accelerates at age 50 – a process known as *sarcopenia*. Exercise actively protects and builds up your lean muscle mass and prevents this process from occurring. Neglecting exercise will only result in a decline in muscle mass – our bodies begin to require fewer calories, our metabolisms slow, and the lost muscle is replaced by fat. Simply put, the amount of muscle mass we have is the primary determi-nant of metabolic rate so we need to hold on to it.

When you start out on your IWL plan don't get disheartened if you don't see the weight decrease on the scales. Statistically speaking, you are likely to fall into that 70 per cent of the population who don't do enough exercise for your general health, so even if you're not losing weight your body is still benefiting from the exercise. To exercise to lose weight, you have to do more than the moderate 2.5 hours a week to just stay alive and healthy.

You need to view exercise as a medicine. For example, I love running. I love the feeling of running fast on the grass and the satisfaction that comes with it, and consequently look forward to exercising every day. Swimming is also a great form of exercise (it's low impact and there are aerobic and strength benefits), but I personally don't like it. So, guess what? I don't do it – it's not for me!

Physical activity activates the brain's pleasure circuit. Exercise will boost your serotonin levels, improving your mood and social functioning. Better still, it will prevent impulsive food choices. What I am telling you is that if you can get your exercise routine into gear everything else will fall into place. You will learn to love exercise and look forward to it. Exercise needn't follow strict routines; anything that gets you moving is just fine.

Do I have to join a gym?

The most important thing is to participate in physical activities that you enjoy, to exercise with others and to explore different environments. Don't go to places you dislike. Some people don't like gyms because it makes them feel bad that they're not as slim as other people there (or fit, strong, or toned) and it reduces their sense of self-worth. Don't join a gym thinking that the expense of membership will coax you into attending. Many of my patients have done this and most of them have found that two weeks after signing they stop going, though they continue to see money being deducted from their account. By all means visit a gym to see if you like it. Some people find that they love it. If you try a range of gyms or fitness centres you may be able to find one that is right for you. Many gyms offer a free trial and many offer a good peer support network where you can discuss your challenges with like-minded people or find training buddies.

On the other hand, if it's not for you, simply walking allows you to be in your natural surrounds. There is not a town, a village or a city where a human being cannot walk and be at peace with themselves. The IWL plan has no interest in getting people to partake in activities that are painful and not enjoyable. If you aren't interested in joining the gym, then do whatever it is that you prefer.

Don't make excuses

We are all busy. Don't make excuses for not exercising, just do it. Finding a minimum of 30 minutes per day for structured exercise adds more than 30 minutes a day to your productivity. It's a net gain which is even more relevant for those who are too busy to exercise. Several of my patients have found that sleeping in their exercise gear gets them up and going first thing, with no time to change their mind. Don't knock it till you try it!

The first thing you need to do is get to the recommended level to stay healthy and that is the 30 minutes of moderate intensity activity, such as walking, cycling or swimming, on five days per week. This can be broken up into blocks of 10 minutes if you have very little time or your joints can't cope. The best type of exercise is walking, cycling or swimming when first starting out. You certainly shouldn't embark on a strenuous exercise routine if you haven't exercised for a while as you are putting yourself at risk of potential heart attack. Start gradually. A health screen at your general practitioner/primary-care provider is strongly advised before starting any type of regime.

Monitoring your activity

The best way to monitor your activity is with a wearable device, a pedometer, or an activity tracking device that can be found on your smart phone. It really doesn't matter what it is, all that matters is that you use one every day of the week. Apple market a watch that is a comprehensive activity device, but it does come with a big price tag. There are devices that can measure water-based exercise or activities other than walking and running, which are great. Most smart phones also measure daily steps, although you have to keep the phone with you for that to work.

Another option is to buy a simple pedometer you can wear on your waist. Cheaper pedometers will certainly have an element of inaccuracy but this does not matter as the over-estimation of your activity level will be consistent every day. Most pedometers work on a ball-bearing technology, meaning that every time you shake them they will record steps regardless of whether you have been moving or not (for example, swivelling on your chair). The over-estimation may be as much as 20 per cent per day, which just needs to be taken into consideration when monitoring your steps. If it says 12,000 steps, it may only be 10,000.

An 'accelerometer pedometer' is a much better choice as it is more accurate and only records movement when you have been moving for more than eight steps or four seconds, and hence is unlikely to over-estimate your day's steps. However, the biggest limitation with a pedometer or accelerometer pedometer (as opposed to a wearable such as a Fitbit or Apple watch) is that you have to clip it to your waist rather than being able to wear it on your wrist. It also won't allow you to measure activities such as cycling, rowing and swimming.

When monitoring your activity on your IWL plan you need to get to 10,000 steps per day, which is the level you should be able to sustain every day of the week. As with your body weight, this is also something that needs to be written down and reflected on at the end of each week. Some days will be a little less but others will be more. As long as the average is 10,000 steps per day over the course of the week, this will ensure you are looking after your health. The 10,000 steps should be met by making sure you incorporate incidental activity wherever you can. Include these tips where practical for your lifestyle:

1. Use the stairs instead of the lift.

2. Take 10-minute breaks from your desk, at least three times per day.

3. Park further away from your workplace to incorporate walking to and from your car.

4. Get off one bus stop earlier than your usual stop.

5. Get public transport instead of driving.

6. Walk or cycle to the shops.

7. Take phone calls while walking around.

8. Use social catch-ups as an opportunity for exercise – instead of going to the coffee shop or the pub, meet your friends for a kick-around or a stroll.

9. Park at the back of the car park to make you walk further to the shops or workplace.

10. Trial a walking meeting.

Find what works for you

You need to establish what works for you, and some people are busier than others. For example, Matt, a current member of the IWL community, is a full-time lawyer at a corporate law firm in the Sydney CBD. He works on average from 8 am to 9 pm every day and it's not unusual for him to be in the office past midnight. He has very little spare time but he has successfully changed his lifestyle and now incorporates the IWL plan as part of his daily life. He walks a part of the way to and from work, runs at lunchtime, plays social touch football once per week, and sets reminders on his phone to move away from his desk at regular intervals every day. His life motto is now 'always take the stairs'. He also spends a few hours on a Sunday night cooking healthy and sustainable meals he can take with him to work throughout the week. There are no excuses!

The 10,000-step goal

Once you have developed a sustainable and realistic habit of 10,000 steps per day (or 60 minutes of leisurely cycling or swimming, which is the equivalent), you should give yourself a pat on the back. This is a huge achievement. Depending on how you are achieving your 10,000 steps will determine whether it is enough to help you lose weight. If it is largely being achieved through incidental activity this is fantastic as it means you are far from sedentary. But, due to the nature of the intensity most likely being low to moderate, it is unlikely to result in you achieving weight loss. If, on the other hand, it's through moderate and vigorous activities and you sweat every day, you may see the weight loss you are after.

The sweat factor

YOU NEED TO SWEAT! If you are sweating every day when you exercise, you are working at the right intensity to lose weight. A patient of mine would always say 'sweat is fat crying'!

I often find that people are confused by what is meant by 'vigorous' exercise. Put simply, if you are sweating, you are doing it right. Vigorous doesn't mean going out for a run or lifting big weights, it could be riding on a stationary bike in the comfort of your own home in front of the TV, if you are getting up a sweat and your heart rate is high.

If you are achieving your 10,000 steps per day (or equivalent movement from cycling or swimming) predominantly from structured rather than incidental activity, you are probably relying on structured activity to achieve your goal and are likely to be very sedentary in your day-to-day life. The problem here is, if you don't keep up the structured activity, you will find you are barely moving at all. This is often seen in people who adopt the all-or-nothing approach, which is not healthy, not sustainable and not advised. If that sounds like you, work out how you can increase your movement, firstly, without the reliance on structured activity – after all, it's not always practical to take a few hours out of your day for structured activity time.

Incidental activity

The first step with your activity on the IWL plan is to increase your activity level through incidental activity. It may take a few months to get to the optimum level of incidental physical activity, and that is fine and advised. It is all about making gradual but realistic and sustainable changes that become a way of life. The gradual increase in your incidental activity level – for example, by initially walking for 10 minutes per day and building up to 30 minutes per day over the course of a month – will also ensure you don't end up injuring yourself or exacerbating joint pain from excess body weight. People often embark on their exercise journey only to be shot down by injury or pain caused by doing too much, too soon. Take it easy and keep the long-term goal at the front of your mind. Sometimes less is more and if you develop an injury it will only set you back further.

If you are not currently performing any activity, the 10,000 steps per day goal (or equivalent movement in cycling or swimming) can also be part of your wash-out period, which we discussed in Chapter 3. You need to allow yourself to get to an incidental activity level that becomes habitual and easy to incorporate into your daily routine.

Once you have adjusted your way of life to focus more on movement you can then start to work on what is required to achieve the small amount of weight loss (approximately 0.5 kg) required per week on the IWL plan. It might simply be the addition of a small amount of structured activity like a social game of soccer or a gym class on top of the 10,000 steps per day, or a change in the type of activity you are doing to get to your 10,000 steps. It's only when you start to do something on top of the 10,000 steps or completely mix up your routine that you will see the weight-loss results you are after. And it's not a matter of doing the same thing every day. Mixing up your routine really is the key to success. I recommend you vary the type and intensity of activity to 'shock' your body into a state of weight loss. The body is very stubborn and won't budge from its state of equilibrium unless a stress is imposed on it. The 'stress' I am referring to here is *variety* rather than anxiety!

Exercise during weight-loss months

During the weight-loss months of the IWL plan it is important to change your exercise routine on a continual basis. This means trying new walking or running routes, working at higher intensities by incorporating hills, or trialling new exercises or activities you have not done before (for example, at the gym, or alternative sports). The higher intensities can be performed on any equipment – bike, rower, or in the pool. You should work at higher intensities for short periods, followed by rest periods to get your breath back. For example, 30 seconds where you work hard, followed by two minutes to allow your heart rate to decrease, and repeating until you can complete a 15–20 minute session.

The variety of activity during the weight-loss months should not be confined to the type of exercise alone. It also applies to where you are exercising. I'm referring to the physical location – the streets you are walking on, the ovals you are training at, and the people you are exercising with. Every time you exercise somewhere different you gain a new energy that you didn't know existed and a new excitement. Every blade of grass, every inch of concrete and every square metre of a fitness centre will offer something that the previous place didn't, and this is the stimulus that you need to stay motivated and achieve the results you are after.

The overall goal with weight loss is to maintain as much of your muscle mass as possible and to see the weight loss coming predominantly from fat stores, which is another key reason why you will succeed long term with the IWL plan. Inevitably you may lose a small amount of muscle mass as well, but the more you can hold on to the better, as muscle is much more metabolically active than fat, meaning it burns more energy at rest and prevents your metabolism from decreasing. The more you preserve your metabolism the easier it is to keep the weight off long term. In other words, the more muscle mass you have, the more calories you will burn.

Exercise during the weight-maintenance months

The great thing is that the weight-maintenance months (every second month) allow you to do the same type of activities, to forget about the variety, and to be less diligent. They allow you the flexibility to take part in less vigorous activities, or less activity in general, to ensure you maintain your weight and prevent it from going down. The weight-maintenance months can be your 10,000 steps per day with light activities, but it does depend on how much you wish to increase your consumption of treat foods or takeaway foods during these months (see Chapter 7 on what to eat) as to how much you can taper down your activity level. You don't need to be sweating it out during the weight-maintenance months, you just need to keep moving.

What should I do if even walking is too much for my joints?

You are not alone in your struggle with this common problem. A large percentage of the population experience joint pain and many patients in my clinical studies have been affected by it.

Excess body weight will impose undue stress on joints, which is exacerbated by certain exercise. If this is the case for you, most incidental exercise will not be practical and you will *only* be able to achieve the recommended amount of physical activity through the incorporation of non body-weight-bearing exercise like cycling and rowing.

Swimming is another great exercise that takes the stress off your joints. It doesn't matter what you do in the pool, all that matters is that you move around and enjoy it.

Don't forget to track your activity even in the water. Many activity monitors these days are waterproof, but if you are using a pedometer or similar device that you can't take in the pool, the general rule of thumb is that 20 minutes of moderate activity equates to approximately 3000 steps.

If you're too self-conscious to exercise in public, aim to include cycling in small, frequent bouts on a stationary bike in the convenience of your own home. Once your weight starts to drop and you alleviate some of the pain and take the stress off the joints, you will find that walking becomes easier and you will gradually be able to increase your activity by incorporating more incidental exercise – a crucial step on your weight-loss journey.

CHAPTER 11

WHAT TO DO IF YOUR WEIGHT ISN'T GOING DOWN

'Courage is knowing what
not to fear' – *Plato*

If you are not seeing any change on the scales during the weight-loss months, this could be due to many reasons. The common ones to look out for are:

1. Not eating five meals per day – skipping meals regularly only to overeat at the next meal.

2. Failing to plan your day – overlooking the importance of scheduling every day (the night before or the morning of).

3. Failing to use a 'to do' list – not writing things down as they pop into your head.

4. Not eating enough – not seeing the weight change on the scales and restricting food intake as a result.

5. Not making sure the majority of your food intake is at the start of the day – failing to make breakfast the biggest meal of the day only to overeat in the afternoon and evening.

6. Eating too fast – not eating with chopsticks or away from technological distraction.

7. Eating when not hungry – forgetting to have a glass of water before every meal or before each sensation of hunger, particularly after dinner.

8. Not eating at the dinner table and away from technological distraction.

9. Not having enough plant-based meals.

10. Lack of exercise variety – it must be completely different to your weight-maintenance months.

11. Not hitting 10,000 steps per day.

12. Too many 'treat' foods – more than one per week.

13. Lack of sleep – less than 6 hours per night.

14. Dining out or getting takeaway too often – more than once per week.

15. Not making the time to prepare evening meals – less than six days per week.

16. Going to bed too late – staying up after 10 pm in front of the TV.

17. Watching TV and mindlessly snacking, scrolling through social media – more than one hour per day.

18. Not using a device to monitor your activity level – neglecting to write down your steps or electronically tracking your activity every day.

Use this checklist as a prompt every time you commence a weight-loss month. If you are convinced that you are successfully putting all of these strategies into practice and you still don't see the weight budging on the scales, don't be alarmed. The last thing you should do is reduce your food intake thinking that is the cause of your problems. Often it is the opposite, and you may actually need to focus on increasing the amount of wholesome and nutritious food you eat (see the list in Chapter 7). This is as long as you are keeping the less nutritious white, refined sources of carbohydrate (including all those foods we think are healthy, like muffins and banana bread) to an intake of once per week.

I would suggest making use of a food journal for at least a month to make sure you are keeping the 'treats' to a minimum, that you are having five meals per day, that you are substituting many of your meat-based meals with legumes or eggs as the protein source, and that you are focusing the majority of your food intake at the start of the day. Pay particular attention to monitoring after-noon and evening snacks. You might find that you are still subconsciously eating after dinner when you are not even hungry. Worse still, it may not be the healthy foods that you are advised to snack on (see Chapter 7).

When recording in a food journal, make sure you do the following:

1. Highlight when 'treat' foods appear in your journal. If it is currently five per week, reduce to four treats, until you work your way to one per week on the weight-loss months. Don't eliminate the treat foods altogether.

2. Count the number of meals per day from breakfast through to dinner. Dessert is not included in this count as very rarely will you need it if you follow the IWL plan properly. You must have five meals per day.

3. Highlight the number of meat-based meals you are consuming. Not every meal needs to contain meat, and by including more vegetarian and plant-based options you will improve your gut microbiome (the healthy bugs in your gut).

4. Record your hunger scale before and after meals to ensure you are seeing a decrease in hunger before meals towards the end of the day. This will only happen if you eat the majority of your food at the start of the day.

-1	0	1	2	3	4
Full and uncomfortable	Not at all hungry	Satisfied	Slightly hungry	Somewhat hungry	Hungry

Above is a hunger scale that you can use. If you notice that your hunger is still higher before meals at the end of the day (a '3' or '4' on the hunger scale), you still have a lot of work to do. Your body hunger signals don't change overnight, especially if you have been doing the same thing for decades (i.e. skipping breakfast and eating little throughout the day, only to have your biggest meal at the end of the day). This takes time to change, but if you do change your food structure and intake you will start to wake up hungrier in the morning and you will feel better for it. You should start to wake up in the '3' range. If you wake up in the '4' range you are doing very well.

After a meal, your hunger should never be in the '-1' range, unless of course it's a one-off like Christmas Day. Very rarely should you even be recording a '0' after a meal. Instead, the majority of the time you should feel '1' after eating, which implies you are satisfied that you have had enough but you do feel like you could eat more food. This is particularly relevant at the end of the day. Once you master your hunger signals and structure of food intake throughout the day you are well on the way to getting into a weight-loss phase. But it can take a while to work out the distinction if you have been eating until you're not at all hungry for years. Remember the 66 days to break a habit rule I told you earlier? Well, this applies here too!

If after keeping a journal you are still convinced that your eating is in accordance with the IWL plan and your weight is staying the same, patience is the key. I implore you not to panic. We WILL get you into a weight-loss phase! It's just that our bodies are very stubborn and cleverly calibrated. They have learnt to become smarter and smarter over time and their job is to resist change or weight loss.

One person who wrote to me about this very problem was a woman I'll call Lauren. She wrote:

Hi, I started your plan a month ago. Despite being super careful about eating the foods (probably eating lots of nutritious food but not enough of it) and exercising most days, I haven't been able to shift any of the weight. After a month on your plan my weight fluctuated from 92.9 to 92.1 but then ended back at 92.3 (0.6 kg loss over the month). Why haven't I been able to lose the 2 kg over the first month?

In this instance, it was Lauren's exercise plan that needed significant change. Despite making some alterations to her food intake, her exercise had stayed the same – in fact, she had been doing the same exercise routine for years. This didn't mean she had to increase her activity level to kick into a weight-loss phase but instead

116

vary the type of exercise she was doing, as well as incorporating a range of different exercise intensities throughout the week. An activity monitor helped Lauren achieve this goal. Encouraging her to never deprive herself of food was also a large part of her success.

In this example with Lauren, she was supposed to be in a weight-loss month when she wrote to me. I suggested she let the month go and focus on weight maintenance for the following month, but keep all aspects of the IWL plan in play.

When the third month began (the next weight-loss month) I told Lauren to completely change the type and intensity of physical activities she was doing. This was the necessary change to see Lauren lose the 0.5 kg per week and resulted in 2.2 kg over the month. To give you an idea of the type of activities she had been doing in the month she didn't lose weight, they were as follows:

Monday	Tuesday	Wednesday	Thursday
Gym – 1-hour yoga session	Pool swimming 20 laps freestyle	1-hour walk on same route around neighbourhood	Pool swimming 20 laps breaststroke
Friday	Saturday	Sunday	
Rest	Gym – 1-hour yoga session	Gym – 1-hour body combat class	

After the change in exercise routine, which saw Lauren kickstart her weight loss, she began doing the following activities (notice the change in days she was doing each type of activity, the change in intensities of each activity, and the change in type of exercise):

Monday	Tuesday	Wednesday	Thursday
Pool swimming 10 laps freestyle – one lap fast, recover for 2 minutes, repeat	1-hour walk stopping at six hills along the way and running up each hill, and recovering at the top	Gym – 30 minutes weight training session using a program provided by the gym instructor	Pool swimming 10 laps breaststroke fast, followed by 10 laps freestyle easy
Friday	**Saturday**	**Sunday**	
Rest	Gym – 1-hour yoga session (change of class to try a different instructor)	Gym – 1-hour class she had never tried before	

Lastly, if you are convinced that your food intake and activity routine is in accordance with the IWL plan, focus on getting more sleep, or at a minimum going to bed earlier and reading until you fall asleep – not looking at your phone! Sleep plays a vital role in weight management and the more you can get the better off you will be. If you are already going to bed early but failing to drift off, use the evening time for constructive activities on your 'to do' list, but try to avoid technology as this can disrupt your circadian rhythm and make it hard to get to sleep.

CHAPTER 12

HELP! MY WEIGHT'S GOING DOWN WHEN IT SHOULDN'T!

'Everything flows, and nothing abides,
everything gives way, and nothing stays
fixed' – *Heraclitus*

It's a wonderful feeling to see the weight coming off the scales, but you still need to ensure you follow the key principles of the IWL plan by putting on the brakes every second month. Never under any circumstance continue with weight loss during a weight-maintenance month. Your body will start to work differently and you will fail long term. Every second month your body needs to rest and re-calibrate its new set point (approximately 2 kg lighter each time).

Many of my patients would get excited by the number on the scales, see the weight coming off and try to lose more. But at around the 2–3 kilogram weight-loss mark, the point considered clinically significant in a medical setting, their body would start to react differently and slow down its functioning. This happens to everyone and I believe that it can be prevented by:

1. Losing no more than 2 kilos per month.

2. Ensuring you give your body a break every second month by not allowing any further weight loss to happen.

If your weight is going down during the weight-maintenance months unintentionally, this could be due to many reasons. The good news is that it is an easy problem to fix and allows you to really take the accelerator off and relax. I stress that it is a problem and must be fixed – you must stop further weight loss from occurring. More than likely you are being overly restrictive with your food intake or not allowing yourself to enjoy your favourite 'treat' foods enough. Don't restrict your food intake; keep the same food plan in place as the weight-loss and weight-maintenance months but allow an extra treat or two – a total of three treats per week on the weight-maintenance month instead of two. You can also allow an extra dining-out or takeaway meal, bringing you to a total of three per week on the weight-maintenance months instead of two. Following the IWL plan will be easy if you don't adopt the all-or-nothing approach that has always failed you in the past. If you stick to the plan and maintain your weight every second month you WILL succeed.

Relax!

The other thing to be conscious of is your exercise routine. This month is not about sweating it out. Remember, this is the month when you can relax a little and do the same thing. You shouldn't add new exercises or different types of exercise, especially if you successfully lost weight the month prior. Just keep the same routine you had in place for the previous weight-loss month but with a shift in intensity to low- to moderate-exertion activities. You don't want to be guilty of doing too much exercise.

Some of my patients who have never dieted or tried to lose weight in the past find that the weight still comes off following a relaxed plan during the weight-maintenance months. This is because a body will always respond faster to weight loss the first time around. If you find yourself in this situation and you are already allowing extra treats and you are not varying your exercise routine or increasing the volume of exercise, you will need to adjust your food intake. Specifically, you will need to include more 'good' fats in your daily eating plan. This means cooking with more olive oil than usual, putting more avocado on your toast, on your sandwich or in your salad, or having two to three times the amount of nuts and seeds that you usually have. These sources of fat are good for our heart health and the best way to increase your calorie intake to ensure you don't keep dropping weight.

As you will come to see, it is not realistic to assume you will have a perfect weight trajectory over any given month. At the end of your weight-maintenance month the goal is to have kept within 1 kg of the previous month's weight. If your weight is down by 1 kg at the end of the weight-maintenance month, factor this into your next month's weight loss, which would mean allowing another 1 kg (and not 2 kg) weight loss in the month that approaches. If your weight is up by 1 kg, factor this into next month's weight-loss goals – aim to be 3 kg down at the end of the weight-loss month. It is a realistic goal to keep within a kilo of your goal trajectory each month due to the huge variance that you see in body weight.

CHAPTER 13

WHAT TO DO WHEN YOU'VE REACHED YOUR GOAL WEIGHT

'We are what we repeatedly do. Excellence, then, is not an act but a habit' – *Will Durant*

Well done! You have reached your realistic goal weight loss. You should be VERY proud of yourself.

The IWL plan doesn't leave you in the lurch once you've reached your goal. Instead, the focus switches as per the instructions and guidelines for the weight-maintenance months. You continue to put everything into place that you have learnt – the new eating habits, regular exercise, using your time productively, and better sleep. And you keep monitoring your weight each week to ensure it stays the same. You never stop following the IWL plan as it becomes a lifestyle, but you can now take the focus off any further weight loss. If you do that you will keep the weight off for life. The old habits won't creep back in because you will have been on the plan for long enough to form a habit. For example, if your goal weight loss was 10–12 kg, you would have been following the IWL plan for a year. Now it's a way of life.

What about those who want to set a new goal weight?

In some instances, you have achieved the realistic goal weight loss that I helped you calculate at the start of the book. You feel great but still want to lose more.

Think back to the case study in Chapter 4, in which Petra's set point was 95 kg and her goal weight loss was 8 kg. This meant her new goal set point was 87 kg. Eight months later Petra successfully achieved the 8 kg weight loss (approximately 2 kg weight loss every second month). She then continued following the weight-maintenance months of IWL from months 8 to 12 and she was comfortably able to maintain this weight loss. Petra was feeling terrific, but after 12 months asked me whether it would be practical and realistic to aim for more weight loss. We reviewed her previous dieting and medical history again and it was achievable to set a new weight-loss goal. In this instance we set another 4 kg to a new set point of 83 kg.

Petra went on to successfully lose this additional 4 kg over the next four months and has maintained her weight loss for more than eight years. She continues to put the

IWL lifestyle into place every day and loves her new way of life, her enjoyment of food and passion for exercise.

Sneaky weight gain

If you notice your weight creeping up (more than 1 kg per year), don't suddenly start to restrict the amount of food you eat as you did in your old dieting days. It just means you need to reflect on a few aspects of your lifestyle. Perhaps you need to reinstate some of the key principles of the weight-loss months such as exercise variety and, in particular, intensity and type of exercise. You also need to reflect on your food intake to see how often you might be eating those treat foods, dining out or neglecting to make breakfast the most important meal of the day. Keeping a food journal will help you assess this as well as your hunger scale before and after meals. Most importantly, it is imperative to keep tracking your weight and recording your steps on a spreadsheet every week.

What are the key aspects of successfully keeping the weight off long term?

1. Continuing to track your body weight each week and monitor the trend over time. If your weight goes up by more than a kilogram over the year, you need to reinstate the aspects of the IWL plan weight-loss months.

2. Revisiting your exercise routine every quarter to ensure you are not doing the same thing day in, day out. You should change what you are doing so that you continue to enjoy your exercise routine and challenge your body with a new stimulus.

3. Keeping a food journal every second month for a period of seven days to ensure you monitor your consumption of treat foods and frequency of dining out. It also allows you to reflect on your hunger scale throughout the day to make sure you are still eating your largest meal at the start and smallest meal at the end of the day.

4. Moving! It doesn't matter what you do as long as it's regular and part of your daily routine. Wearing a device that tracks your activity is a great way to keep an eye on it.

5. Cooking enough food every night so that you have enough for lunch leftovers the following day. Most people don't have enough time to cook or prepare every meal so make things easy for yourself.

CHAPTER 14

FREQUENTLY ASKED QUESTIONS

'The only true wisdom is in knowing you
know nothing' – *Socrates*

Since the release of *Interval Weight Loss* I have compiled a list of the things I've been most commonly asked, but if you have a question that isn't covered here I'd encourage you to get in touch through the 'Dr Nick Fuller's Interval Weight Loss' Facebook page. Please do not hesitate to reach out if you are uncertain about anything as this will ensure you succeed on your IWL plan.

Is all sugar bad for you?

Since books about quitting sugar became popular, there has been much confusion about what constitutes a sugar and the difference between each type of sugar. Do not let someone convince you that because a food contains 'sugar' it is bad for you. Added sugars and naturally occurring sugars are not the same thing. Many foods contain naturally occurring sugars and these foods are very good for us (for example, fruit and dairy). They are excellent sources of nutrition and important for our long-term health.

On the other hand, added sugars are the bad sugars and you will find them predominantly in food products coming out of a packet, such as snack bars, or white refined carbs such as pastries, confectionary and sweets. As a general rule of thumb, food in its natural form may contain sugars that are naturally occurring and good for us, and food coming out of a packet may contain added sugars that are not good for us.

Does sugar cause diabetes?

Sugar in foods does *not* cause diabetes. Type 1 diabetes is an auto-immune disease (there is no cure and it can't be prevented) and carrying excess body weight is a risk factor for type 2 diabetes. Foods that contain added sugar, such as pastries, chocolate, ice-cream, or anything that is processed and comes out of a packet, are high in energy. If you regularly eat these foods it is likely you will be consuming too many calories and put on weight, and could develop type 2 diabetes down the track.

Ingredients to watch out for when looking for added sugars on labels include:

Brown sugar

Corn syrup

Fruit juice concentrates

Glucose solids

High-fructose corn syrup

Invert sugar

Malt sugar

Molasses

Raw sugar

Sugar

Sugar molecules ending in 'ose' (e.g. dextrose, glucose, sucrose, maltose, fructose).

Doesn't fruit have sugar and therefore need to be avoided?

Yes, fruit does contain sugar but these are naturally occurring sugars. Fruit or other foods containing naturally occurring sugars do not make us fat or cause diabetes, but it is best to limit your intake of juice or dried fruits as they are concentrated sources of sugar and calories.

If I buy skim or low-fat milk will it have added sugar?

Skim/no-fat or low-fat milk will not have added sugar. The only difference between full-fat and the low-fat or skim alternatives is that the fat is literally skimmed off the top of the milk. Skim or low-fat milk will have the same protein and calcium without the high fat content.

What about yoghurt?

You do need to be a little careful with yoghurt. To keep things simple, choose one that says 'no fat' *and* 'no added sugar' on the label.

Does low-fat dairy include low-fat yoghurt?

Yes, but low-fat or no-fat yoghurt can also have added sugar. The easiest way to know what to choose in the supermarket is to go for the 'low-fat' natural yoghurt or a 'no-fat' yoghurt that also specifies that it has 'no added sugar'. The no-fat or low-fat dairy option has the same nutrition as full-fat but with half the energy.

Is the IWL plan for everyone?

I have had countless enquiries about whether the IWL plan can be followed by people of different ethnicities and cultural eating patterns. Yes, absolutely! It can be followed by anyone. The IWL plan is an adaptive approach that can be tailored to your lifestyle. If you're a vegetarian, take the meat out. If you're allergic to salmon, don't make the salmon recipe.

Is the IWL plan suitable for those with diabetes?

Yes, it is most certainly suitable for those with diabetes – both type 1 and type 2. It is important, however, that if you have diabetes and take glucose-lowering medications or insulin, you discuss the IWL plan with your doctor before starting. If you have type 2 diabetes, losing weight may help prevent the disease from progressing further and in some instances may help you get rid of the disease altogether. It is also suitable for those with insulin resistance or pre-diabetes as the weight loss you will achieve may get your body working properly again and prevent your developing the disease.

Is the IWL plan suitable for those with food intolerances?

Yes, if there is a particular recipe that includes milk, for instance, and you are lactose intolerant, you will need to substitute it with a lactose-free alternative, such as lactose-free milk. Similarly, those with coeliac disease will need to find a replacement for a product containing gluten or eliminate it. If you are diagnosed with lactose intolerance or coeliac disease and are still unsure which ingredients are suitable substitutes, please make contact through the Facebook page for some suggestions.

Is the IWL plan suitable for vegans or vegetarians?

Yes, most certainly. Again, simply substitute any meat products with suitable alternatives. For example, meat with tofu, or chicken with beans.

Can the IWL plan be followed by those with hypothyroidism or an under-active thyroid?

Yes, however it is *vital* to follow up with your general practitioner regarding your medication and dosage and ensure your thyroid function is regularly monitored with a blood test. Weight loss may alter your thyroxine requirements and therefore your medication may need adjusting as you progress on the IWL plan.

Can the IWL plan be followed by those on medications for depression or other mental disorders?

Yes, but you should follow up with your general practitioner if you suspect weight gain due to the particular medication/s you may be taking. There is a greater availability of approved medications for treatment of depression and mental disorders nowadays that do not have a negative effect on body weight, and these may be applicable to your specific condition.

Is the IWL plan suitable for those with cancer or in remission from cancer?

Yes. More and more cancers are being linked to obesity so eating foods such as wholegrain carbohydrates, fruits and vegetables can only help. Please be aware, of course, that if you have cancer you will still need treatment.

Apart from my body weight, what else should I be measuring?

You should have your height accurately measured so you can calculate your BMI. The BMI is your weight over your height squared. There are lots of online calculators that you can use after you accurately measure your height and weight for the first time. One suitable example is found at: www.healthdirect.gov.au/bmi-calculator. The BMI should be used in conjunction with waist circumference. BMI reference points for males and females are:

Under 18.5	Underweight
18.5–24.9	Healthy weight range
25.0–29.9	Overweight
30.0 +	Obesity

You can also monitor your waist circumference, your radial pulse and your blood pressure. The waist circumference should be measured by someone else to ensure an accurate measure. For consistency, the most accurate point of reference is the belly button. Ensure the tape measure is square around the waist when the reading is taken. For females work towards a goal waist measure of less than 80 cm and for males less than 94 cm.

Your pulse can be taken on the radial artery, located on the lateral side of the wrist (just under the attachment of the thumb). The average normal pulse rate for males and females is 60–80 beats per minute. Athletes tend to have recordings of 40–60 beats per minute. If your pulse is above 100 beats per minute at rest you should visit your GP for a health screen.

Lastly, your blood pressure can be taken with a digital machine that you can purchase from a pharmacy or department store. Ensure you are seated, have been resting for a few minutes, and that you are not talking when the measure is taken. A normal reading for males and females is 120/80. If it is above 140/90 you should visit your GP for a health screen.

Where do I go for further help? Can I get face-to-face consultations?

Unfortunately I am not taking on further patients at this time but you can engage with me on social media. The good news is that you do not need face-to-face contact to succeed on the IWL plan. People most benefit when they read the book more than once – the more times the better to help instil the principles and core understanding of the

IWL plan. Write down the 'do's and don'ts' provided at the back of this book and stick the list on your fridge or in your diary as a gentle reminder. The foods that you need to eat on the IWL plan should also be written down and the list stuck on your fridge so that every time you are hungry you are reminded what you can eat. This is exactly what it is designed for. Lastly, don't hesitate to ask a question at the 'Dr Nick Fuller's Interval Weight Loss' Facebook page where there is a community of people following the IWL plan, or at the www.intervalweightloss.com.au website.

Can I substitute dishes/recipes with my own favourites?

Yes, absolutely. The daily meal and monthly plans are just a guide. This book is not intended to be a cookbook but rather give you some good ideas on what you can make, how easy it can be to cook using just a few ingredients, and to show you what ingredients you should use as the foundations for recipes. When following the IWL plan you don't need to rely on meal plans, count calories or weigh out portions of each ingredient. You can put any of your favourite recipes into the weekly food plan if they are based on the core principles of the IWL plan. Just remember the following:

- Cook with raw ingredients.
- Cook with olive or canola oil only (the occasional teaspoon of sesame oil or other oil is fine).

- Include plenty of vegetables or salad vegetables with each recipe (including with pasta-based meals).
- Ensure you include a protein source and a wholegrain carbohydrate source with each recipe to ensure your daily meal plan is nutritionally balanced and contains all the core food groups at each meal.

How do I know how much to eat?

There is very little in my books and meal plans about exact quantities to eat. This is intentional because it is *not a diet* and you won't succeed if you rely on a set eight-week plan, 12-week plan or similar.

We all need guidance but it's up to you to learn how much to eat at each meal by listening to your body signals and by ensuring that you eat a lot at the start of the day and very little at the end. For most, this will mean completely switching around the structure of your current food intake. When I mention oats for breakfast, load up your bowl on the first few occasions because breakfast is the most important meal of the day and should be the biggest (but you can split it up into two smaller breakfasts – one before work and one when you arrive at work). If you can't get through the portion or feel uncomfortably full at the end of the meal, you have eaten too much and you need to reduce the quantity the next day until you master it. This is because everyone needs a different intake and males will usually need more than females (sometimes 1½ times the intake) as they have a larger body mass.

The same applies for dinner. If a particular recipe specifies how many it makes or how many it serves, this is a guide so that you can make an appropriate amount to also factor in leftovers for the next day's lunch. One such example is Family-favourite Spaghetti Bolognese (page 199), which can be made in a large batch.

There is no exact portion size and you will learn to appreciate how much food you need for each meal. A great tool to use is the hunger scale provided earlier and at the back of the book. This is particularly helpful when first starting the IWL plan to continually assess how hungry you are before and after each meal.

The meal must also be balanced. Half the meal should be vegetables or salad, with a quarter being a wholegrain carbohydrate source such as a piece of bread or serving of rice, and a quarter being your protein source such as meat, fish or lentils.

What size should my evening meal be?

Your evening meal should fit onto a bread-and-butter-sized plate or a small rice-sized bowl. A rice bowl is a small bowl used in Asian cuisine for rice. It's the perfect tool for measuring out your evening meal. If you are hungry after having this small portion for dinner you should wait 10 minutes before considering going back for a second portion. In this instance, you may need to start eating more food at the start of the day to ensure you are less hungry by the time dinner comes around. And don't forget your chopsticks!

Is it bad to eat late at night?

It is not always practical to have an early dinner. Eat dinner when you can but make sure it is the smallest meal of the day. This is even more important when having your evening meal later in the evening as you are less likely to wake up feeling hungry if you overeat at night.

I never wake up hungry. What should I do?

It takes time for your hunger cues to change and if you have been doing the same thing for years or decades (i.e. skipping breakfast because you're not hungry) your body's signals will not change overnight. Coffee can also alter or mask your appetite, so make sure you have something with your morning cuppa. If you have changed your meal orientation to ensure you are having your smallest meal at dinner you are well on the way to success and you will start to wake up feeling hungrier. Just give it time!

Are products such as Weet-Bix and All-Bran cereal products considered packaged food?

Despite coming out of a packet you can rely on break-fast cereal products that are based largely on wholegrain wheat. However, it is important to bear in mind that these products will also contain other added ingredients such as salt and sugar, and there are more suitable breakfast options such as oats, avocado on wholegrain toast, or fruit and yoghurt.

Which milk is best?

Cow's milk is the richest source of calcium, protein and iodine. If looking for a dairy-free and lactose-free alternative to cow's milk, calcium-fortified soy milk is the next best option from a nutritional perspective. Rice milk and almond milk are low in protein.

Can I eat any type of nuts and seeds?

Yes, you can enjoy a range of nuts and include a mix, including walnuts and almonds. Choose dry-roasted or in their natural form, without added oil or salt.

Are activated almonds better than normal almonds?

No, they are exactly the same. 'Activation' does not improve the digestibility and nutrition of the nut, despite the clever marketing.

Can I drink soda water in place of water? Does soda water have sugar?

You should focus your fluid intake on water and have soda water when dining out (it makes you feel like you are treating yourself to something other than alcohol). Soda water does not contain sugar but it does contain sodium, so don't have it as your primary source of fluid. Even mineral or sparkling water can contain sodium, depending on the brand, so be sure to check what you're buying if you're drinking it every day. And for those who drink tonic water, remember this is a treat too as it also contains sugar. If you must have it then stick to the 'diet' option.

Is it bad to eat carbs at night?

No, I suggest you eat carbs with every meal. Choose the wholegrain types and this will ensure every meal is balanced and help you feel fuller for longer. There is no research to suggest that carbs at night make you put on weight.

Should I take supplements? If so, which ones?

If you are eating all of the foods suggested in this book you will *not* need supplements. This includes multivitamins. If you are a vegan, however, or attempting to fall pregnant, there are certain supplements that you should take. Vitamin B12 will be needed if you are avoiding all animal products and you should consult with your general practitioner for a subcutaneous injection or appropriate supplement.

How do I lose the weight off my tummy and hips?

This is referred to as 'spot reduction' and unfortunately there is no such thing. Those late-night TV ads promising to shrink your stomach are all lies. You can't lose weight in one specific spot. When you lose weight it comes off the entire body. Your body will continue to change over time on the IWL plan but don't expect your tummy to disappear from doing lots of crunches or sit-ups. The tummy, hips and thighs are the most stubborn areas of all and often the last to see change.

Should I exercise in the morning or evening?

Exercise when it suits you. It doesn't matter when you do it; all that matters is that you do it.

Will weights make me big?

No, weight or resistance training adds variety to your exercise routine and will not result in you putting on weight or gaining bulky muscle.

Is there any way you can download the weight-loss chart provided at the back of the book?

Yes, this can be downloaded from www.intervalweight-loss.com.au.

What should I be eating during the maintenance period? Do I just eat the same way I have been eating during the weight-loss month but eat more dinner?

You should structure your food intake in the same way during the maintenance periods as the weight-loss months – largest meal at breakfast and smallest meal at dinner. You should not be eating more at dinner. The maintenance months allow you the flexibility to include more of those treat foods you love or to eat out more regularly. For a detailed explanation of how to adjust your eating plan in the weight-maintenance months, refer to Chapter 7.

What should I do if my weight isn't going down during the weight-loss month?

A step-by-step guide is provided in Chapter 11 so you can get to the root cause.

What about other weight-loss programs such as keto, Paleo, 5:2 and intermittent fasting? Are they any good?

Please refer to the first chapter for a detailed answer to this commonly asked question. Everyone talks about these diets at the moment due to clever marketing but the research is not there to back them up. Intermittent fasting is *not* the same as Interval Weight Loss.

If a program is commercially available and large scale does this mean it can be trusted?

No, many of the weight-loss programs and products that are now available do not even have evidence to back up their claims. This includes commercial weight-loss programs. Many of these commercial providers just use testimonials and case studies on their websites for how much weight people lose. This is not real research – this is anecdata – and anyone can post such claims. With respect to the commercial programs that provide all your meals, you may lose weight at first as you are eating meals that are calorie controlled, but as we all know, it is not realistic to stay on this food forever. We get bored of it, it's expensive and repetitive, and it's not a sustainable or educational approach to being healthy or long-term weight loss.

CHAPTER 15

CASE STUDIES

'Time is the wisest counsellor of all' – *Pericles*

The following are real-life case studies of people who are currently part of the IWL community and on the IWL plan.

CASE STUDY 1 – JACQUELINE

I am 57 and since my late forties have started gaining more weight than I'd like. I followed a low-carb Bodytrim system and lost 10 kg within a year or so. I kept the weight stable for a little but have been gaining ever since. I am a vegetarian, but have been eating fish as well for many years now. I was born and bred in Italy, so growing up the Mediterranean diet was my staple. But since the Bodytrim days, I have cut down on all carbs and increased my plant-based protein intake. I always use low-fat or no-fat dairy (rich, fatty foods make me queasy).

I do 11,500 steps a day and work out three days a week. I read in your book that I should vary my workout routine. I am organised and task-oriented but still gain weight and am currently 88.4 kg, the highest I've ever been. Can you help me, please?

Scenario:

As predicted, Jacqueline's weight has been increasing since stopping the low-carb diet she was following and she is now at her highest body weight/set point. The biggest hurdle will be trying to get Jacqueline to reintroduce healthy wholegrain carbohydrate foods as she is still restricting carbs. I also suspect she may be restricting her food intake and not eating enough. She is doing a lot of exercise and is most likely aerobically fit and healthy, which is great.

Advice:

1. Reintroduce wholegrain carbohydrates to ensure a nutritionally balanced food plan is being followed for Jacqueline's long-term health and weight management.

2. Change the food structure to make sure Jacqueline is having the majority of her food intake at the start of the day and the least amount at the end.

3. Ask Jacqueline to monitor her hunger scale throughout the day and to observe whether she is comfort eating at various times, noting it in a food journal.

4. Advise her to increase her food intake from wholesome, nutritious foods and to allow occasional treat foods to ensure she is not being overly restrictive.

5. Encourage Jacqueline to change her 'workout' days, try new exercises and activities, and incorporate a range of intensities of varying durations – this doesn't mean Jacqueline needs to do more exercise.

6. If time permits, incorporate an extra day of structured activity and something different to the exercise she has been doing in the past.

CASE STUDY 2 – JEFF

Hi, I have just bought your book and read it over the weekend. I am quite sedentary in my job and will be starting to walk for 45 minutes a day again after not being active for a while due to severe plantar fasciitis (heel pain). I also enjoy yoga, but I don't think these exercises will be enough to comply with your suggestion of being more active and counteract all the extra food I will be eating. Can you provide some suggestions, please?

Scenario:

Jeff suffers from a condition called plantar fasciitis, meaning he gets inflammation and pain in the heel and arch of the foot. It is most likely that this flares up when he starts an exercise routine or is doing too much without the necessary preventions in place. There is no information provided on his food intake so we can only focus on his exercise routine in the first instance.

Advice:

1. Start by walking 10 minutes a day and ensure Jeff builds this up gradually over the course of a month until 30 minutes per day is achieved. Forty-five minutes is too much to commence with, especially as Jeff has a previous history of plantar fasciitis.

2. It is important that Jeff does a non body-weight-bearing exercise every second day such as swimming, rowing or bike riding to ensure he alleviates the stress on the tissue and ligaments of the foot.

3. If any pain in the arch or heel of the foot becomes evident it is important for Jeff to ease off and focus his activity only on non body-weight-bearing exercise (swimming, riding or rowing).

4. Get Jeff to perform some specific prevention exercises to release the plantar fascia of the foot, such as standing barefoot on a hard ball and rolling it under the arch. This should be done daily for a couple of minutes on each foot.

5. Once Jeff is confident that the plantar fasciitis is no longer a problem, he can mix up the type of physical activity and start to include more variety in the intensity of exercise.

CASE STUDY 3 – HELEN

I started this plan two months ago. I am only 5 feet tall and started at 62.9 kg. I am enjoying the food. This was no surprise to me as I used to restrict my carb intake and then binge occasionally on certain carb foods. It took me a few weeks to understand and trust in you that carbs are okay. I have always exercised before starting this plan. Despite exercising most days I haven't been able to lose any weight. After two months my weight has varied from 62.8 to 62.2 kg. It went down as low as 62.0 kg. Is this fluctuation normal? Should I be concerned about the lack of weight loss? Should I continue on the weight-loss month until I reach 2 kg or should I commence my maintenance month?

Scenario:

It is important to realise that Helen does not have much weight to lose when referring to a crude measure (BMI). Based on the measures provided, her BMI is 27.1 kg/m². It also appears she has a history of dieting/following fad eating principles as she has been restricting her carb intake for an unknown period of time. It is likely that the reintroduction of carbs would have seen an increase in her weight due to water content. Remember, this is not an increase in fat mass. Helen also mentions that she regularly exercises.

Advice:

1. Ensure weight has stabilised after the reintroduction of carbohydrate foods. This might take several weeks. Once it has stabilised, aim for 1 kg weight loss per month rather than the normal 2 kg as starting weight/BMI is not high.

2. Ask Helen to also measure and monitor her waist circumference as this will provide a more comprehensive assessment of her health.

3. Wear a trackable device to monitor activity level. Despite exercising regularly, Helen's incidental activity may not be high.

4. Completely change Helen's structured exercise routine to include new activities and a range of activities at different intensities throughout the week.

5. Do not continue with weight loss during the maintenance periods. It is important to only aim for the 1 kg weight loss every second month and to allow the body to rest between these weight-loss months.

PART 2

CREATIVE COOKING

You should now have all the knowledge you need to succeed on the IWL plan. This next section of the book is intended to provide you with some examples of the types of meals you can include on the IWL plan. It is not intended to be a cookbook, but rather give you some ideas of what you can cook, how easy it can be using just a few ingredients, and show you which ingredients you should use as the foundations for recipes. With technology and social media platforms at our fingertips, there is never a shortage of recipes that can be adapted to your IWL plan.

A recipe is suitable if it includes raw ingredients, olive or canola oil only (the occasional tablespoon of sesame oil or other oil best suited to a specific cuisine is fine), plenty of vegetables or salad, a protein source and a wholegrain carbohydrate source. There are times when convenience foods do play a role, such as pastry or stock, but cooking can be just as easy when using raw ingredients rather than pre-made ones.

Cooking is a wonderful and fulfilling aspect of a healthy lifestyle as it encourages us to appreciate and enjoy food. Not only will it ensure you are eating better, it will also save you money. It can be very easy if you stick to just a few ingredients and recipes that don't take all night to cook. Refer to the *Store Cupboard Essentials* at the end of the book to ensure you have all the core staples to hand. You shouldn't have to spend all afternoon at the supermarket looking for obscure ingredients and you shouldn't need to be in the kitchen all night cooking. No one has time for that. Everyone can learn the basics of cooking – it just takes a little practice. And it can be every bit as easy if you have children as they can be part of the cooking experience, which will in turn teach them important life skills.

I have included serving sizes for each recipe, but please note that they are not gospel and are simply there to give you a guide. You need to serve your evening meal on a bread-and-butter-sized plate or in a small bowl and have the leftovers for lunch the next day (lunch will be a larger portion). Breakfast will be your largest meal and dinner the smallest, with lunch somewhere in between. Adjust the quantities of each recipe to ensure you cook extra at each evening meal as this will go a long way towards ensuring success on your IWL plan. You should always have leftovers as this takes the pressure off having to prepare or think about lunch when you wake up in the morning. It's also a vital step of successful meal preparation to ensure you don't rely on trying to find healthy takeaway options for lunch each day.

Even if you have never tried cooking, give it a go. It is a key to success and designed to be simple on the IWL plan.

FRESH VEGETABLES AND HERBS

There's a lot to be said for growing your own vegetables and herbs, and you don't need a big garden to do it. Some of the best veggie gardens I have seen are grown on cleverly configured green walls in small apartments. Having your own veggie garden doesn't require much effort and just a little maintenance will go a long way to ensuring an ongoing supply of fresh produce is at your fingertips. The only exception is if your place doesn't get any sun.

The core staples of any basic garden should include rosemary, basil, parsley, shallots, coriander and rainbow spinach or another green leafy vegetable such as kale, baby spinach or rocket. Mint is also a handy one to grow as it's good for warding off bugs and flies. Be careful though as it behaves like a weed and can take over your entire veggie garden. Coriander is the most challenging herb to grow, but the others will often thrive with some sunlight, water and good nutrient-rich soil. Don't buy the cheap potting mix as it will ensure failure!

Picking your own fresh produce is extremely satisfying and growing everything from seed can save a lot of money. (Tomatoes in particular are easy to grow and you will notice they taste much sweeter than those you get from the supermarket.) Think about all the times we buy fresh and expensive herbs from the supermarket, only to use a small quantity and see the rest go to waste. Having your own veggie garden is also a great way to involve your children. Handing them this responsibility gives them a sense of contribution to the family meal when they go to pick the crops.

Your local nursery is an excellent starting point to help work out what you can grow in your home environment. Start small and expand your collection of herbs as you gain understanding about what grows best and at what time of the year. For those who find they have a green thumb, the range of growing opportunity is endless.

BREAKFAST

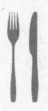

OVEN-BAKED NUTTY MUESLI

This is a great recipe that you can make in any quantity and use for breakfast throughout the week. Scoop it into a bowl each morning, then add your choice of milk and a large spoonful of blueberries. Delicious!

This recipe will make enough to fill a large Tupperware container to use for breakfast throughout the week.

3 tablespoons cashews
3 tablespoons almonds
small handful of pistachios, shelled
3 tablespoons walnuts
2 cups (180 g) steel-cut oats
1 tablespoon ground cinnamon
1 teaspoon vanilla extract (not essential)

1. Preheat the oven to 180°C and line a large baking tray with baking paper.
2. Using a mortar and pestle, lightly pound all the nuts together (this step is not compulsory and you can simply add the nuts as they are).
3. Spread out the nuts and oats on the prepared baking tray and sprinkle over the cinnamon and vanilla extract.
4. Bake for 15–20 minutes or until you can smell the cinnamon.
5. Allow to cool completely, then store in an airtight container for up to 2 weeks.

MISO SCRAMBLED EGGS WITH VEGETABLES

Miso eggs are a delicious way to add variety to your weekend hot breakfast. The miso adds a delicious extra flavour and makes the whole dish taste better. Try using one teaspoon of miso paste the first time as the flavour can be quite intense. You can add some short-cut bacon to this breakfast recipe occasionally to make it an even more filling and wholesome meal.

Serves 4

6 eggs
2 generous teaspoons miso paste (white or yellow variety is
    preferred)
olive oil spray
large handful of silverbeet, finely chopped
2 large mushrooms (portobello or similar), finely chopped
leftover vegetables (if you have any), finely chopped
½ avocado
4 slices wholegrain bread, toasted

1. Crack the eggs into a bowl and whisk with the miso paste.
2. Spray a large frying pan with olive oil and heat over medium heat. Pour in the egg mixture and cook, stirring, for 3 minutes or until cooked to your liking. Transfer the scrambled eggs to a large bowl and cover with foil to keep warm.

3. Add the silverbeet and mushroom to the pan, along with any leftover veggies or bacon (if using) and spray again with olive oil. Cook for 3–5 minutes.

4. Toast your wholegrain bread and then spread the avocado evenly over each slice. Top with the scrambled eggs, silverbeet, mushroom, bacon (if using) and any other vegetables.

Tip: The miso will be easier to whisk into the egg if it is at room temperature rather than straight out of the fridge. I sometimes run the packet under warm water to heat it up a little.

Fun fact: Eggs are a complete protein source and, despite being high in cholesterol, will not raise your blood cholesterol. You can enjoy up to 12 eggs per week. Yes, that's right, 12 eggs a week, as long as you are not loading them up with bacon, butter and all the usual ingredients that go with a big fry-up!

CINNAMON FRENCH TOAST

Cinnamon is a spice that comes from the bark of several different tree species. It is a versatile ingredient and has a delicate though sweet and woody flavour that can be utilised in both sweet and savoury dishes, making it a wonderful addition to so many foods and recipes.

Serves 4

4 eggs
2 teaspoons ground cinnamon
8 slices wholegrain bread
olive oil spray
300 g raspberries or blueberries (fresh or frozen)
honey, for serving

1. Crack the eggs into a bowl and whisk in the cinnamon with a fork.
2. Soak each slice of the bread in the egg mixture.
3. Heat a large frying pan over medium heat. Spray with olive oil. Add the bread to the frying pan in two batches and cook on each side for 2 minutes.
4. Serve with berries and a drizzle of honey on top.

BAKED BEANS

These baked beans can be enjoyed as a main or side dish. They go particularly well with eggs on some freshly baked wholegrain bread from your local baker. I love to make them on a Sunday. I make myself a coffee, pick up the paper, and have the perfect start to my day.

Serves 2

1 tablespoon olive oil
½ brown onion, finely chopped
1 x 400 g tin roma tomatoes, chopped
1 x 400 g tin red kidney beans, drained and rinsed
2 teaspoons honey
pinch of sea salt
2 teaspoons finely chopped coriander

1. Heat the olive oil in a saucepan over medium heat. Add the onion and cook for 3–5 minutes or until softened.
2. Add the tomato and cook for a further 10 minutes or until the tomato breaks down and the mixture becomes a sauce.
3. Add the beans, honey and salt. Reduce the heat to low and cook for a further 10 minutes.
4. Stir in the coriander, then serve and enjoy.

BREAKFAST ON THE GO

This is a great smoothie to prepare the night before an early start, ready to grab out of the fridge in the morning. It's not enough to have by itself but it is a great option on busy mornings. Make sure you complement the smoothie with something more substantial, such as some muesli, after arriving at your workplace. On less busy mornings it's better to have a more solid start to the day and to try some of the other breakfast recipes. Remember that calories from a juiced or blended liquid are not as satiating as eating the whole food.

Serves 1

3 dates, pitted
boiling water, to soften
½ banana
1 cup (250 ml) skim milk
1 teaspoon tahini

1. Place the dates in a small cup or heatproof bowl, cover with boiling water and leave to soften for 1–2 minutes. Drain.
2. Transfer the dates to a blender, add the remaining ingredients and blend until smooth.

Fun fact: A large glass of juice will typically have 2.5 times the energy content and one-third the fibre content of a piece of fruit. A smoothie has even more – the additional ingredients mean it will have around 4 times the calorie content of a piece of fruit, so whenever you can, opt for the whole fruit instead. To read my full story on juicing, please go to www. intervalweightloss.com.au.

BERRY AND BANANA PANCAKES

A word of warning before you start: these pancakes are absolutely delicious but they do require a lot of patience as they need to be cooked over very low heat. Both sides will need at least 5 minutes to cook through. A good tip is to use two frying pans, which will cut the total cooking time in half.

Serves 4

150 g almonds

3 bananas

3 eggs

160 g blackberries, raspberries or blueberries (thawed if frozen)
    + extra for serving

¾ teaspoon baking powder

1½ teaspoons ground cinnamon

honey, for serving

olive oil spray

1. Place the almonds in a blender and pulse to a flour consistency.
2. Mash the bananas in a large mixing bowl. Crack the eggs into the bowl and mix well.
3. Add the blended almonds, berries, baking powder and cinnamon and mix well.

4. Spray the large frying pan with olive oil (or two frying pans if you have them) over medium heat (you will be required to spray the pan with olive oil after cooking each batch of pancakes).

5. Reduce the heat to low and pour the pancake batter into the pan. The smaller you make them, the easier they will be to turn. Cook for about 5 minutes or until they don't stick to the spatula when you attempt to flip them. Flip them over and cook for another 5 minutes or until golden and cooked through. Transfer to a plate and cover to keep warm while you cook the remaining pancakes. Serve with berries and a drizzle of honey on top.

Tips: You can buy almond meal but it is cheaper to buy almonds and blend them to an almond meal yourself.

Blackberries, raspberries and blueberries all work well in this dish. Unless the berries are in season, opt for the frozen packets as they will be cheaper.

SOUPS AND SALADS

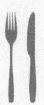

PESTO-INFUSED POTATO, ZUCCHINI AND LEEK SOUP

This recipe calls for pesto – ideally homemade (see my recipe on page 244) but you can use good-quality bought pesto if you don't have time to make your own.

Don't get too caught up if you are missing a couple of the ingredients listed below. Just use whatever vegetables you have in your fridge or garden – soup is a great way of using them up. The same goes for the soup mix; if you only have lentils or split green peas, they will be just fine.

There is a flavour difference between the white and green part of a leek. The green has a strong taste, which is fine to include if you like bolder flavours, but I usually save it for making homemade stock.

Serves 4

2 garlic cloves, finely chopped

1 cup (200 g) split green peas

1 cup (220 g) soup mix

½ leek, white part only, washed and chopped

handful of kale leaves, chopped

handful of rocket, chopped

4 zucchini, cut into bite-sized pieces

1 cup (120 g) frozen peas

2 potatoes, peeled and cut into bite-sized pieces

1 stick celery, finely chopped

small handful flat-leaf parsley, finely chopped

1.25 litres vegetable stock
freshly ground black pepper
pesto (see page 242), to serve

1. Turn your slow cooker on low. Add the garlic, split peas, soup mix, vegetables, parsley and stock.
2. Season with pepper and cook on low heat for 3–4 hours. (You can also put everything in the cooker last thing at night and allow it to cook overnight, then turn it off first thing in the morning – it will be fine to simmer away for 6–10 hours.)
3. Stir in a dollop of pesto just before serving.

Tips: As with all the soup recipes, a saucepan can be used if you don't have a slow cooker. A slow cooker, however, is a wonderful asset in the kitchen. You will find yourself reaching for it quite often, especially during the colder months. They also save a lot of time as you simply chop up all the ingredients, add them to the slow cooker and then leave to simmer away on a low heat for 6–10 hours overnight. Voila! You have a delicious soup ready in the morning when you get up.

If using a saucepan, just make sure you prepare the vegetables and begin cooking as soon as you get home from work. It can then simmer for a couple of hours while you unwind or take care of other household tasks. Bear in mind, though, that a longer cooking time will bring out the full flavour of each of the soups.

ANDREW'S WHOLESOME VEGETABLE AND BEAN SOUP

This is my brother's favourite hearty winter soup. He would always make it on his designated day of cooking in the family when we were growing up. A longer cooking time is preferred for this recipe as it allows the soup mix to soften and combine well with the other ingredients.

Serves 8

1 brown onion, finely chopped
1 garlic clove, finely chopped
1 carrot, chopped
1 large potato, peeled and chopped
1 stick celery, chopped
1 sweet potato, peeled and chopped
500 g soup mix
1 litre vegetable stock, plus extra if needed
1 x 400 g tin cannellini beans, drained and rinsed
1 x 400 g tin whole tomatoes (tinned or diced tomato varieties are also fine to use)

1. Turn your slow cooker on low and add all the ingredients. Ensure there is enough liquid in the cooker – if it appears vegetable-heavy with very little liquid, add some more stock or water.
2. Cook overnight on low heat for 6–10 hours.

SLOW-COOKED PUMPKIN SOUP

Pumpkins are one of the most popular foods, and one doesn't have to guess why; they are extremely cheap and they taste great. They are also very versatile and keep for ages. The only con is that they're challenging to cut, so watch out for your fingers. Look for one that is firm (it shouldn't give when you press into the skin) and heavy for its size. It should have a consistent colouring on the skin. Personally, I love the butternut variety as it has a sweet-tasting flesh which is perfect for soups.

Serves 12

1 tablespoon olive oil
3 brown onions, finely chopped
4 garlic cloves, finely chopped
2 kg pumpkin (any variety is fine), peeled, seeds removed and
    roughly chopped
1 teaspoon ground cumin
2 litres vegetable stock
sea salt and freshly ground black pepper
finely chopped flat-leaf parsley, to garnish

1. Turn your slow cooker on low heat.
2. Heat the olive oil in a frying pan over medium heat. Add the onion and garlic and cook for 2 minutes, then remove from the heat and add to the slow cooker.

3. Add the pumpkin, cumin and stock, and season with pepper and a pinch of salt.

4. Cook on low heat for 6 hours or until the pumpkin is soft.

5. Cool slightly, then add to a blender (or use a stick blender) and blitz until smooth.

6. Serve topped with a sprinkling of parsley.

SWEET POTATO, TOMATO AND CHICKPEA SOUP

As with the majority of the IWL soup recipes, this is another very simple recipe to cook overnight in a slow cooker on low heat, which takes away the burden of having to keep an eye on the stove for a couple of hours when using a saucepan.

Serves 4

1 brown onion, chopped finely

2 garlic cloves, crushed

3 baby eggplants (or 1 large eggplant), cut into bite-sized
    pieces

1 medium sweet potato, peeled and cut into bite-sized pieces

1 zucchini, cut into bite-sized pieces

freshly ground black pepper

1 x 400 g tin whole or chopped tomatoes

1 x 400 g tin chickpeas, drained and rinsed

1 litre vegetable stock

2 tablespoons finely chopped flat-leaf parsley

olive oil, for cooking

1. Heat some oil in a frying pan and add onion and garlic. Cook on medium heat for three minutes, or until lightly browned.
2. Turn your slow cooker on low heat.
3. Transfer all the vegetables to the slow cooker and add the tinned tomatoes, chickpeas and stock.

4. Cook on low heat for 6–10 hours (this soup will be sufficiently cooked after 3 hours if you are pushed for time).
5. Using a potato masher, mash the mixture together. Stir in the chopped parsley, season with black pepper and serve.

AARON'S VEGGIE LENTIL SOUP

This is a family friend's favourite recipe that regularly appears on our weekly food plan. As with most of the soups in this chapter, it makes a large batch that you can use for leftovers throughout the week or freeze for quick weeknight meals.

Serves 8

1 brown onion, finely chopped
1 garlic clove, finely chopped
1 stick celery, finely chopped
1 carrot, cut into bite-sized pieces
1 medium potato, peeled and cut into bite-sized pieces
1 x 400 g tin brown lentils, drained and rinsed
2 x 400 g tins whole or chopped tomatoes
1.5 litres vegetable stock
1 tablespoon tomato paste
1 tablespoon soy sauce

1. Turn your slow cooker on low and add all the ingredients.
2. Cook overnight on low heat for 7–9 hours.

HALOUMI, BEETROOT AND QUINOA SALAD

Beetroot has an earthy yet slightly sweet flavour, making it a wonderful addition to salads. They are a rich source of fibre and potassium.

Beetroot is delicious both roasted and steamed; however, I'd recommend putting on some gloves when cleaning and cutting them due to their staining potential. For steaming, simply chop them up into quarters or eighths and leave the skin on. Steam for 20 minutes above some boiling water. Once they are cooked and tender, allow to rest and cool before rubbing off their skin with your fingers.

If roasting, preheat oven to 180°C, and clean and peel the beetroot. Cut them into bite-sized pieces as this will reduce the cooking time, and add them to a baking tray sprayed with olive oil. Roast for 20 minutes.

An even simpler and more convenient option is to buy the vacuum-sealed pre-packaged beetroot which is 100 per cent beetroot. This is also delicious and cuts down on a lot of mess and cooking time for this recipe.

Serves 4

1 cup (190 g) quinoa (see Fun fact)
2 potatoes, peeled and diced
1 tablespoon olive oil
125 g (half a regular-size packet) haloumi cut into bite-sized pieces
6 baby beetroot or 2 large beetroot, cooked and cut into
    bite-sized pieces

1 continental cucumber, cut into bite-sized pieces
2 large handfuls of baby spinach leaves
1 avocado, diced

1. Cook the quinoa according to the packet instructions.
2. Meanwhile, place the potatoes in a small saucepan, cover with water and bring to the boil. Cook for 5 minutes or until tender. Drain.
3. Heat the olive oil in a frying pan over medium heat and cook the haloumi until golden.
4. Tip the cooked quinoa into a large salad bowl, add the potato and scatter the haloumi over the top.
5. Add the beetroot, cucumber and spinach leaves to the salad bowl and gently toss to combine.
6. Top with the diced avocado and serve.

Fun fact: Pronounced 'keen-wah', quinoa is an extremely versatile wholegrain with a rich, nutty flavour. It's also a wonderful source of protein, so next time you don't feel like rice or couscous, opt for quinoa instead.

FALAFEL-STYLE SALAD

This salad is a great way to enjoy everything you love about falafels without actually having to make them. It's quick, easy and delicious.

Serves 4

1 cup (190 g) quinoa
handful of flat-leaf parsley, roughly chopped
handful of coriander, roughly chopped
1 x 400 g tin chickpeas, drained and rinsed
125 g cherry or grape tomatoes, quartered
50 g Danish feta, crumbled

Tahini dressing
¼ cup (65 g) tahini
1 garlic clove, finely chopped
3 tablespoons lemon juice
½ teaspoon ground cumin
1 fresh chilli, finely chopped
pinch of sea salt

1. To make the dressing, place all the ingredients with ¼ cup of hot water in a small blender and blend until smooth and well combined.
2. Scoop the dressing into a bowl and place in the fridge until needed.

3. Cook the quinoa according to the packet instructions. Tip into a bowl and allow to cool.
4. Add the parsley, coriander, chickpeas and tomato to the quinoa.
5. Spoon the dressing over the salad and gently toss to combine.
6. Scatter the feta over the top and serve.

Tip: Wrap the salad in a freshly baked wholemeal Lebanese bread and toast in a sandwich press for a wholesome and filling lunch.

CAULIFLOWER RICE, CHICKEN AND CASHEW SALAD WITH LIME DRESSING

Cauliflower is not always the most popular of vegetables in our household but making it into 'rice' is a fun and delicious way of incorporating more vegetables into the IWL eating plan. It's easy to make at home – all you need to do is grate it into pieces approximately the size of rice grains. Here we boost the protein content with some grilled chicken.

Serves 8

1 large head cauliflower
3 tablespoons olive oil
500 g chicken breast or thigh fillet, trimmed and cut into
    bite-sized pieces
2 teaspoons grated ginger
⅓ cup (80 ml) lime juice
1 tablespoon soy sauce
2 small red chillies, finely chopped
large handful of kale, roughly chopped
1 red capsicum, seeds and membrane removed, chopped
1 cup (150 g) cashews (dry roasted or natural)
1 cup coriander leaves or rocket, roughly chopped

1. Using the medium holes of a food grater, 'rice' the cauliflower. This should yield about 5–6 cups.

2. Heat 2 tablespoons of olive oil in a large frying pan over medium heat, add the cauliflower rice and cook for 5 minutes, stirring frequently. Transfer to a bowl and allow to cool.

3. Meanwhile, heat the remaining olive oil in a frying pan over medium heat. Add the chicken and cook for a minimum of 5 minutes or until lightly golden and cooked through, with no pink in the centre.

4. Place the chilli, kale and capsicum into the frying pan with the chicken and cook over medium heat for a couple of minutes or until softened.

5. Combine the ginger, lime juice and soy sauce in a small bowl to make the lime dressing.

6. Add the capsicum mixture, cashews and coriander or rocket to the cauliflower rice. Pour the lime dressing over the top and gently toss to coat. Enjoy!

Tips: This salad does not keep well beyond the day of cooking as it can go soggy. It's best prepared shortly before you are ready to eat.

All nuts are great sources of protein and fat, and peanuts also go very well in this salad. You can read up on the facts about nuts in the weekly articles at www.intervalweightloss.com.au.

SASHIMI BEETROOT SALAD

As with the Haloumi, Beetroot and Quinoa Salad, to steam the beetroot simply chop them up into quarters or eighths and leave the skin on. Steam for 20 minutes above some boiling water. Once they are cooked and tender, allow to rest and cool before rubbing off their skin with your fingers.

If roasting, preheat oven to 180°C, and clean and peel the beetroot. Cut them into bite-sized pieces, as this will reduce the cooking time, and add them to a baking tray sprayed with olive oil. Roast for 20 minutes.

The simplest and most convenient option is to buy the vacuum-sealed pre-packaged beetroot which is 100 per cent beetroot.

Serves 2

2 x 150 g salmon fillets, skin removed (see Tips)
6 baby beetroots, cooked and cut into bite-sized pieces
2 shallots, finely chopped
juice of 1 lemon
2 large handfuls rocket or baby spinach leaves

1. Wash the salmon under running water, then pat dry with some paper towel and cut into bite-sized cubes.
2. Place the salmon in a bowl and add the beetroot, shallot, lemon juice and rocket or spinach. Gently toss to combine and serve.

Tips: The words 'sashimi-grade' and 'sushi-grade' are often bandied about, although they mean precisely nothing. These terms originated for marketing purposes. There is no national governing body that grades fish as it does with beef. Anything labelled 'sashimi-grade' is what the seller has judged as safe to eat raw. The key is to find yourself a good fish retailer, as when it comes down to it, the claim is only as trustworthy as the fish market itself.

If you dislike raw fish (and don't worry, you're not the only one), you can cook it before adding it to the salad. Heat a drizzle of olive oil in a frying pan over medium heat, add the salmon and 1 tablespoon of sesame seeds and lightly sear, turning frequently, for 2 minutes.

POKE BOWL

Poke bowls (pronounced 'poh-keh') are a popular Hawaiian dish that have been making a name for themselves all over the world. They usually contain raw fish, rice and vegetables and you can make all sorts of variations on the one below. They are a fun meal to share with others as you can cut up all the ingredients and leave them in individual bowls for everyone to pick and choose their preferred combination. A poke bowl is a fresh and simple way to add variety to your eating plan.

Serves 2

2 x 150 g salmon fillets, skin removed (see Tips in 'Sashimi Beetroot Salad' on page 186)
1 x 250 g packet pre-cooked brown rice (you can also cook rice from scratch but this is just a quick option on time-poor nights)
1 cup (220 g) kaleslaw (see Tips)
⅓ cup (65 g) red cabbage sauerkraut (see Tips)
½ avocado, cut into bite-sized pieces
1 Lebanese (short) cucumber, diced
2 tablespoons sesame seeds
1 tablespoon fried shallots (you can buy these at the supermarket)
sriracha sauce (see Tips), to serve (optional)

1. Wash the salmon under running water, then pat dry with paper towel and cut into bite-sized cubes.
2. Cook the rice according to the packet instructions.
3. Place the rice in a bowl and add the salmon, kaleslaw, sauerkraut, avocado, cucumber, sesame seeds and fried shallots. Gently toss to combine and serve with sriracha sauce, if desired.

Tips: Kaleslaw (a combination of shredded vegetables including kale, red cabbage, parsley, dill, green shallots and carrot) can be bought pre-made in the supermarket. The same goes for the red cabbage sauerkraut used in this recipe – this can also be bought pre-made in the supermarket. Alternatively, try the recipe on page 246.

Sriracha is a type of hot sauce or chilli sauce made from a paste of chilli peppers, distilled vinegar, garlic, sugar and salt. You will find it in most major supermarket chains or your local Asian supermarket. And if you can't find it, this recipe goes well with any hot sauce.

MAIN MEALS

BEEF, CARROT, POTATO AND CABBAGE STEW

During the winter months, our food preferences change.
To prevent comfort eating, a wholesome, hearty stew is the
ultimate warming meal. The main difference to a soup is the
consistency; stews have a thicker texture and when done right,
as with this recipe, they are a very healthy and filling meal, and
an easy way to increase your vegetable intake. Don't forget
to use your chopsticks, or if that's too challenging try using a
teaspoon so you don't wolf down your meal.

Serves 8

2 tablespoons olive oil
1 brown onion, finely chopped
1 carrot, chopped
1 potato, chopped
3 garlic cloves, finely chopped
500 g lean beef mince
4 cups (1 litre) vegetable stock
1 large shredded white cabbage, core removed
2 x 400 g tins whole or chopped tomatoes
large pinch of dried oregano
handful basil leaves, finely chopped
large handful kale leaves
large pinch freshly ground black pepper
1 tablespoon lemon juice
small handful finely chopped flat-leaf parsley

1. Heat the olive oil in a large heavy-based saucepan over medium heat. Add the onion and garlic and cook for 5 minutes.
2. Add the beef mince and cook, breaking up any lumps with the back of a wooden spoon, until lightly browned.
3. Add the stock, carrot, potato, cabbage, tinned tomatoes, oregano, basil and a large pinch of pepper. Cover and bring to the boil, then reduce the heat to low and cook gently for at least 60 minutes.
4. Mix in the kale leaves and parsley. Serve.

CHICKEN, ROAST PUMPKIN AND SESAME SEED BOWL

Bowl meals are certainly the current craze. Easy, fun and simple to prepare, they are ideal inclusions on the IWL plan as you eat out of small bowls and tend to use chopsticks. Research has shown that simply switching to smaller bowls and plates can prevent overeating.

Trial your own variety and tag us on Instagram @intervalweightloss.

Serves 4

400 g pumpkin, any variety, peeled and cut into small bite-sized
   pieces
olive oil spray
2 large chicken thighs, trimmed and cut into bite-sized pieces
1 small bunch broccolini, cut into thirds
3 tablespoons red cabbage sauerkraut (see recipe on page 246)
Handful of cherry or grape tomatoes, halved
handful of rocket
1 avocado, diced
1–2 tablespoons sesame seeds

1. Preheat the oven to 180°C and line a baking tray with baking paper.
2. Arrange the pumpkin on the prepared baking tray in a single layer and lightly spray with olive oil. Roast for 15–20 minutes or until tender.

3. Meanwhile, spray a frying pan with olive oil over medium heat. Add the chicken and cook for about 7 minutes or until golden brown and cooked through with no pink in the centre.

4. Place the broccolini in a microwave-safe bowl and cook in the microwave on high for 2 minutes or until just tender. The broccolini can also be steamed above some boiling water for a few minutes.

5. Arrange the pumpkin, chicken, broccolini, sauerkraut, tomatoes, rocket and avocado into each bowl and sprinkle with the sesame seeds. Enjoy!

JAPANESE-INSPIRED MISO BEEF WITH EGGPLANT AND BROCCOLI

The best cut of meat for this dish is one meant for grilling or pan frying. Typically, these cuts come from the short loin or sirloin area – areas of the cow that are not tough. They are more expensive, though, so buy according to your budget and try your local wholesaler butcher, where you will find better bargains and better quality meat. Look out for T-bones, porterhouse, sirloin and strip loin. The most tender and expensive cut of beef is the tenderloin.

Serves 4

1 x 500 g piece beef
olive oil spray
1 head broccoli, cut into florets
1 eggplant, thinly sliced
salt
black pepper
chilli flakes, if desired

Marinade
2 tablespoons red miso paste
2 garlic cloves, finely chopped
3 teaspoons sesame oil
2 teaspoons grated ginger
2 teaspoons sesame seeds

1. To make the marinade, combine all the ingredients in a bowl.
2. Rub the marinade all over the beef, place in a glass or ceramic bowl and marinate for 30 minutes.
3. Heat a large frying pan or cast-iron plate over low heat and spray with olive oil. Add the beef to the pan and cook for 10–12 minutes, turning once. Remove and set aside, cover, and allow to rest.
4. Add more oil to the pan, increase the heat to medium, add the broccoli and eggplant and season with salt and pepper, and chilli flakes, if desired. Cook, turning occasionally, for about 10 minutes or until cooked to your liking.
5. When the veggies have been cooking for a few minutes, slice the beef, then cover with foil and rest for another 5 minutes or so. Serve with the eggplant and broccoli.

Tip: Some supermarket chains stock jarred garlic, in its natural form. Look at the ingredients – it should only contain garlic (usually around 88%) and vinegar. Generally, 1 teaspoon is equivalent to 1 clove. This serves as a good back-up that you can keep in the fridge for those occasions when you run out of fresh garlic, but be aware that fresh garlic will always give more flavour to your cooking.

ROAST CARROT AND PUMPKIN WITH HUMMUS AND POMEGRANATE DRESSING

This is a great vegetarian recipe that is very popular in our household. Remember, you don't need meat at every meal and there is plenty you can do to add some flare to a veggie-based dish.

The pomegranate fruit is red, round and looks like a red apple with a flower-shaped stem. The skin of the pomegranate is thick and inedible but there are hundreds of delicious seeds within the fruit. These are a wonderful addition to salads and a great topping on pizzas. This recipe calls for two pomegranates.

Serves 4

250 g butternut pumpkin, cut into small cubes
250 g carrots, cut lengthways into strips
2 tablespoons olive oil
2 tablespoons honey
1 cup (250 ml) Rustic Hummus (see page 237)
70 g pistachios, shelled
seeds of 1½ pomegranates
large handful of rocket
pinch of sea salt

Pomegranate dressing
2 tablespoons lemon juice
1 tablespoon olive oil
seeds of half a pomegranate

1. To make the dressing, whisk together all the ingredients in a small bowl.
2. Preheat the oven to 180°C and line a baking tray with baking paper.
3. Place the pumpkin and carrot on the prepared baking tray, add the olive oil, salt and honey and rub over the vegetables to coat.
4. Roast 40 minutes or until tender.
5. Spread the hummus onto a large serving plate and arrange the roast vegetables on top.
6. Scatter over the pistachios, pomegranate seeds and rocket.
7. Pour over the pomegranate dressing and serve hot.

Tip: To extract the seeds from a pomegranate, cut the fruit in half and place a very large bowl in the sink. Squeeze one half of the fruit at a time over the bowl and the seeds will start to pop out. Use a sharp knife to extract the last few resilient warriors.

FAMILY-FAVOURITE SPAGHETTI BOLOGNESE

Whenever you have a pasta-based dish, serve it with a side salad. This is the Mediterranean way and how pasta meals should be eaten and enjoyed. A simple salad with iceberg or cos lettuce, tomatoes and olives, tossed with some olive oil, balsamic vinegar and dried herbs is the perfect accompaniment to this recipe.

Serves 8

2 tablespoons olive oil
1 white onion, diced
2 cloves garlic, crushed
1 kg lean beef mince
⅓ cup (90 g) tomato paste
2 x 400 g tins whole or chopped tomatoes
2 carrots, diced
4 large handfuls of baby spinach
1 red capsicum, seeds and membrane removed, chopped
1 litre vegetable stock
sea salt and freshly ground black pepper
500 g spaghetti (see Tips)

1. Heat the olive oil in a large, deep frying pan over high heat, add the onion and garlic and cook for 3–5 minutes or until softened.

2. Reduce the heat to medium. Add the mince and cook, breaking up any lumps with the back of a wooden spoon, until lightly browned. Add carrot and capsicum and cook for a couple of minutes.
3. Add the tomato paste, tinned tomatoes, spinach, stock and a pinch each of salt and pepper. Cook for 1 hour or until a thick, rich sauce has formed.
4. Shortly before the bolognese is ready, cook the pasta according to the packet instructions. Drain and serve topped with the sauce.

Tips: The bolognese can also be cooked in a slow cooker. Just put all the ingredients (except the pasta) in your slow cooker on low heat and leave for several hours, stirring occasionally.

Try serving the bolognese with wholemeal pasta, which has roughly twice the fibre content of regular pasta.

DELICIOUS CRISPY-SKIN SALMON WITH GREENS

Salmon is a rich source of omega-3 which is important for brain and heart health, and it reduces inflammation in the body. Try incorporating more fish and vegetarian-based meals in place of meat, especially on the weight-loss months of your IWL plan. Tinned tuna and salmon is a great way to add extra fish to your eating plan and serves as a great snack with crackers, or in a salad.

Serves 2

200 g thin egg noodles
½ teaspoon sesame oil
2 garlic cloves, crushed
2 handfuls silverbeet, roughly chopped
handful of baby spinach leaves
1 head broccoli, cut into florets
2 tablespoons soy sauce
2 teaspoons oyster sauce
olive oil spray
2 x 150 g salmon fillets, skin on

1. Cook the noodles according to the packet instructions. Drain.
2. Meanwhile, heat the sesame oil and garlic in a large frying pan over low heat. Add the broccoli, silverbeet, baby spinach, soy sauce and oyster sauce and cook, stirring regularly, for 8 minutes. Remove from the heat and cover to keep warm.

3. Spray a second frying pan with olive oil and heat over medium heat. Add the salmon, skin-side down, and cook for 5 minutes, then turn over and cook for a further 2 minutes, or to your preference. (Salmon does not need to be cooked through and can be eaten raw.)

4. Serve the salmon on a bed of noodles topped with the greens.

Fun fact: Broccoli is a dark-green, cruciferous vegetable, purported to be a super-food for cancer protection, but ALL vegetables have been associated with cancer-protecting effects and you should be aiming to get in 5 serves per day. To give you an idea, 1 serve is equivalent to ½ cup of cooked broccoli, pumpkin or carrot, or 1 cup of green leafy or raw salad vegetables. Fewer than 5 per cent of the population meet the recommended number of vegetable serves per day. Take up the 5-serve challenge at 'Dr Nick Fuller's Interval Weight Loss' Facebook page.

CRUNCHY CHICKPEA AND MISO BLACK RICE BOWL

This is a versatile recipe as you can use pretty much any combination of vegetables you like. So, don't worry if you don't have any kale or eggplant – just use whatever you have in your crisper drawer.

Serves 2

1 x 400 g tin chickpeas, drained and rinsed
1 teaspoon white or yellow miso paste (see Tips)
1 teaspoon sesame oil
1 teaspoon olive oil
2 baby eggplants, cut into bite-sized pieces
sea salt
large handful of kale
2 eggs
250 g packet pre-cooked black rice (see Tips)
½ avocado, thinly sliced
sesame seeds, for sprinkling (optional)

1. Preheat the oven to 220°C and line a baking tray with baking paper.
2. Place the chickpeas, miso paste and sesame oil in a bowl and stir to combine well. Spread out the mixture on the prepared baking tray and bake for 30–40 minutes or until crisp (watch carefully as they can burn).

3. Meanwhile, heat the olive oil in a frying pan over medium heat. Sprinkle a little salt over the eggplant, then add to the pan with the kale and cook for 5 minutes or until the eggplant is golden. Move the mixture to the side of the pan.

4. Crack the eggs into the pan and fry sunny side up, or to your preference.

5. Cook the black rice according to the packet instructions.

6. Remove the chickpeas from the oven. Divide the rice between two bowls and top with the eggplant mixture, crispy chickpeas, egg and avocado. Sprinkle with sesame seeds if you have them and enjoy!

Tips: You will find white, yellow, red and black miso on the supermarket shelves. The darker the colour, the stronger the taste, so a red miso can overwhelm a mild dish like this. You're much better opting for the milder white or yellow varieties.

Black rice has a nutty, earthy flavour that is perfect for this dish, but don't panic if you don't have it in stock – brown rice will do just as well. Both brown and black rice are higher in fibre than white as they are less processed, meaning they fill you up for longer. You can cook the rice from scratch if you like, but I often find it quicker and easier to use the pre-cooked packets of rice you find in supermarkets.

HEALTHY NACHOS

This version is made with beef mince, but you can easily make it vegetarian by replacing the beef with another tin of red kidney beans.

Serves 8

1 tablespoon olive oil
1 brown onion, finely chopped
500 g lean beef mince
1 x 400 g tin red kidney beans, drained and rinsed
1 red chilli, finely chopped
2 tablespoons tomato paste
1 x 400 g tin whole or chopped tomatoes with Italian herbs
    (or keep it plain if you prefer)
1 x 230 g packet wholegrain tortilla chips
⅓ cup (40 g) grated cheddar
1 avocado, diced
handful of coriander leaves, rocket or kale

1. Preheat the oven to 180°C.
2. Heat the olive oil in a large frying pan over medium heat, add the onion and cook for 3 minutes or until softened.
3. Add the mince and cook, breaking up any lumps with the back of a wooden spoon, until lightly browned.
4. Stir in the kidney beans, chilli, tomato paste and tinned tomatoes. Reduce the heat to low and simmer for 10 minutes or until the mixture thickens.

5. Spread the corn chips across two deep baking trays. Top with the mince sauce and sprinkle on the grated cheese.
6. Bake for about 8 minutes or until the cheese has melted.
7. Top with the avocado and coriander/rocket/kale, and serve.

Tip: If you prefer your nachos crunchy, sprinkle some corn chips on top of the mince sauce as well.

ROAST CHICKEN AND VEGETABLES

Whole chickens can weigh anything from 1.2 kg to 2.5 kg but somewhere in the middle is about right for this recipe. This is a great one for the family to enjoy for a weekend lunch.

Serves 8

1 x 1.8 kg chicken, washed and patted dry
sea salt and freshly ground black pepper
1 lemon, halved
1 tablespoon olive oil
1 sweet potato, peeled and cut into large pieces
100 g pumpkin, peeled and cut into large pieces
4 large potatoes, peeled and cut into large pieces
2 zucchini, cut into large pieces
1 red capsicum, seeds and membrane removed, cut into large
     pieces

1. Preheat the oven to 220°C and line a large roasting tin with baking paper. Place a wire rack in the tin.
2. Season the chicken cavity with salt and pepper.
3. Squeeze the juice of half a lemon over the chicken, rubbing it into the skin. Place both lemon halves in the chicken cavity.
4. Tie the chicken legs together with kitchen string. Brush the olive oil all over the chicken and season with salt and pepper.
5. Place the chicken on the rack in the prepared tin, breast-side up.

6. Scatter the vegetables around the chicken underneath the rack and roast for 60–80 minutes. Season the vegetables with black pepper. As a rule of thumb when roasting chicken, for every kilogram you need to roast for approximately 40 minutes.

7. Remove the chicken and let it rest for 10 minutes before carving. Serve with the roast vegetables.

Tip: Dental floss works as a wonderful back-up if you don't have any kitchen string to truss the chicken – just avoid the mint variety!

KIMCHI STIR-FRY

Kimchi is a spiced fermented cabbage dish and is a staple in Korean cooking. Interestingly, the Koreans have one of the lowest obesity rates in the world. It is often said that while Westerners snack on cheese, Koreans snack on kimchi. It can be purchased from some of the larger supermarkets, but superior varieties will be found in Asian grocery stores. If it's not for you, try replacing it with red cabbage in this stir-fry.

Serves 6

2 teaspoons sesame oil
3 garlic cloves, finely chopped
3 spring onions
2 teaspoons finely chopped/grated ginger
2 teaspoons chilli paste
1 head broccoli, cut into florets
2 large carrots, finely chopped
1 bunch bok choy, leaves removed and chopped, stems diced
1 x 375 g packet egg noodles
150 g firm tofu, cut into bite-sized pieces
4 large mushrooms, cut into bite-sized pieces
2 handfuls of baby spinach leaves
3 tablespoons soy sauce
2 tablespoons oyster sauce
3 eggs
3 tablespoons kimchi (any variety you like)
1 tablespoon sesame seeds
large handful of bean sprouts

1. Heat 1 teaspoon of sesame oil in a deep frying pan or wok over high heat.

2. Reduce the heat to medium. Add the garlic, shallot, ginger and chilli paste and cook for 3–5 minutes or until softened and fragrant.

3. Add the broccoli, carrot and bok choy stem (reserve the leaves for later) and cook for 5–10 minutes or until tender. Remove from the pan.

4. Meanwhile, cook the noodles according to the packet instructions.

5. Heat the remaining sesame oil in the pan and increase the heat to high. Add the tofu and mushroom and cook, stirring regularly, for 6 minutes.

6. Return the vegetable mixture to the pan and reduce the heat to medium. Add the reserved bok choy leaves, baby spinach, and soy and oyster sauces and mix well.

7. Crack the eggs into a bowl and lightly whisk, then add to the pan. The egg will cook through the mixture. Add the cooked noodles and mix well.

8. Just before serving, stir in the kimchi.

9. Garnish with sesame seeds and bean sprouts, and serve.

Tip: I know a lot of people don't like tofu and it is not essential in this recipe. You can replace it with chicken or take it out entirely. The dish will still be nutritionally balanced.

This recipe also works well when substituting the egg noodles with brown rice.

DELICIOUS LAMB SHANKS

This is a wonderful one-pot meal. Toss all your ingredients into a single pan and voila, you have a no-stress, no-mess recipe for any night of the week. This lamb recipe also works well when served on a bed of quinoa with salad if you would rather omit the vegetables.

Serves 4

4 French-trimmed lamb shanks
2 garlic cloves, crushed
1 cup (250 ml) chicken, beef or vegetable stock
juice of 1 lemon
1 teaspoon finely grated lemon zest
2 sprigs rosemary
4 large potatoes, peeled and cut into large pieces
2 carrots roughly chopped

1. Turn your slow cooker on low and add all the ingredients. Cook on low heat for 1½ hours or until the lamb is tender. Alternatively, place all the ingredients in a deep heavy-based saucepan, then cover and cook over low heat for 1½ hours or until the lamb is tender.
2. Divide the lamb shanks and vegetables among serving plates and enjoy.

Tip: Lamb doesn't need to cook right through when served as a whole piece of meat, such as a shank, cutlet or chop. You only need to cook it through when meat is ground or minced. Be aware that lamb has a stronger and longer-lasting flavour than chicken and beef.

QUINOA WITH ROAST ZUCCHINI, PUMPKIN AND PESTO

This vegetarian recipe has some delicious flavours, largely brought about by the addition of cinnamon to the zucchini and pumpkin.

If you don't have any homemade pesto in the fridge, it's fine to use a commercial variety as back-up. Just be aware that it won't have the same flavour or nutrition as a homemade one.

Serves 4

2 large zucchini, cut into large pieces
500 g pumpkin (any variety), peeled and cut into bite-sized
    pieces
2 tablespoons olive oil
1 teaspoon ground cinnamon
½ cup (95 g) quinoa
juice of 1 lemon
2 tablespoons chopped flat-leaf parsley
⅓ cup (90 g) pesto (see page 242)

1. Preheat the oven to 180°C and line a baking tray with baking paper.
2. Place the zucchini and pumpkin on the prepared baking tray, drizzle over the olive oil and sprinkle with cinnamon. Gently toss to coat, then spread out in a single layer.
3. Bake for 30 minutes or until the pumpkin is tender.
4. Meanwhile, cook the quinoa according to the packet instructions.

5. Remove the vegetables from the oven and combine with the quinoa, lemon juice, parsley and pesto.

6. Serve in bowls and enjoy.

Tip: On time-poor days, cut the pumpkin into smaller pieces as this will reduce the cooking time.

BEEF AND ZUCCHINI PIE

Yes, you can still enjoy a pie on the IWL plan! This delicious and nutritious recipe calls for filo pastry (tissue-thin sheets of dough) which in contrast to puff pastry has very little saturated fat, as it is predominantly water and flour. It's a great one for the whole family to cook. And as with many of the recipes in this book, you shouldn't feel that you have to stick rigidly to the vegetables listed below. It's fine to make substitutions according to what you have to hand.

Serves 6

1 tablespoon olive oil
1 brown onion, finely chopped
500 g lean beef mince
1 carrot, finely chopped
1 potato, peeled and finely chopped
2 zucchini, finely chopped
⅓ cup (40 g) frozen peas
125 g cherry or grape tomatoes, halved
1 cup (250 ml) beef or vegetable stock
2 tablespoons wholemeal plain flour
olive oil spray (optional)
4–5 sheets filo pastry
1 egg, lightly beaten

Side serving
2 carrots, cut into bite-sized pieces
1 zucchini, cut into batons

1 sweet potato, peeled and cut into batons
1 potato, peeled and cut into bite-sized pieces
mixed dried herbs, for sprinkling
1 teaspoon olive oil

1. Heat the olive oil in a large frying pan over medium heat, add the onion and cook for 4 minutes or until softened and lightly browned.
2. Add the mince and cook, breaking up any lumps with the back of a wooden spoon, until lightly browned.
3. Add the carrot, potato, zucchini, peas, tomatoes and stock, sprinkle over the flour and cook, stirring regularly, for 3–4 minutes or until the vegetables are tender and the sauce has thickened. Remove from the heat and set aside to cool.
4. Preheat the oven to 200°C. Spray a large round pie dish with olive oil or line with baking paper.
5. While the pie filling is cooling, line a baking tray with baking paper and prepare the vegetables for the side serving. Place the vegetables in a zip-lock bag, add the herbs and olive oil and turn to coat in the oil. Tip them onto the prepared baking tray and spread out in a single layer.
6. Line the prepared pie dish with three sheets of filo pastry. Spoon in the cooled filling, then place the remaining sheets of filo on top. Fold in the overhanging pastry and glaze the top with the beaten egg.
7. Place the pie and side vegetables in the oven and bake for about 30 minutes or until the pastry is golden and slightly crispy and the vegetables are cooked through.
8. Serve and enjoy!

TERIYAKI SALMON SALAD

This is a dish that can be whipped up in minutes and is very easy to prepare. It can also be cooked with either salmon, chicken or beef. If using chicken, opt for breast fillets, and if using beef, try rump steak. Even though it won't be as tender as sirloin steak, it is a much cheaper cut that works well with this recipe. It is also full of flavour. If you use a meat tenderiser mallet before cooking, it will help to break down the muscle fibres and tenderise the meat.

Serves 2

⅓ cup (80 ml) teriyaki sauce
1 tablespoon sesame seeds
4 x 150 g salmon fillets, skin on
1 cup (200 g) brown rice
olive oil, for cooking
½ cabbage, shredded
large handful of baby spinach leaves or kale, roughly chopped
2 carrots, finely chopped
1 head broccoli, cut into florets

1. Combine the teriyaki sauce and sesame seeds in a glass or ceramic bowl. Add the salmon and set aside to marinate for 10 minutes.
2. Meanwhile, cook the rice according to the packet instructions.

3. Heat a splash of olive oil in a large frying pan over medium heat, add the cabbage, spinach or kale, carrot and broccoli and cook, stirring regularly, for 7–10 minutes or until cooked through. Remove to a bowl and cover to keep warm.

4. Wipe out the pan, then pour in another splash of olive oil. Add the salmon, skin-side down, and cook over medium heat for 3 minutes. Turn and lightly sear the other side, then remove from the heat. (Feel free to cook it right through if you prefer.)

5. Scoop the rice onto two plates, add the salmon and finish with the vegetables.

VEGETABLE DHAL

This is not a difficult recipe but it does take a while to cook, so is perhaps best saved for a weekend meal. It's also a great recipe to make in large batches and store in the freezer for emergency lunches.

Serves 8

1 tablespoon olive oil
½ brown onion, diced
3 garlic cloves, finely chopped/crushed
1 teaspoon grated ginger
3 carrots, finely chopped
1 teaspoon ground turmeric
1 teaspoon ground cinnamon
1 cup (200 g) red split lentils
500 g butternut pumpkin, peeled and cut into small pieces
2 tablespoons white or yellow miso paste
handful of coriander leaves
2 tablespoons lime juice
freshly ground black pepper

1. Heat the olive oil in a large frying pan or saucepan over medium heat. Add the onion, garlic, ginger and carrot and cook for 3–4 minutes or until softened.
2. Add the turmeric and cinnamon and cook, stirring, for 1 minute.

3. Reduce the heat to low. Add the lentils, pumpkin and 5 cups (1.25 litres) water and simmer for 1½ hours or until softened.
4. Stir in the miso paste, coriander and lime juice. Season with black pepper.
5. Serve and enjoy!

Fun fact: Foods in the legume family are good sources of protein and have a low glycemic index, meaning they are broken down more slowly in the body, providing energy over a longer period. Lentils and split peas are two such examples, and they can be used interchangeably in this recipe. You can buy them dried (which need to be soaked before cooking) or tinned. Legumes make an ideal protein base for vegetarian or vegan dishes as a substitute for animal products.

CHICKEN SKEWERS WITH ISRAELI SALAD

To make the most of the flavours in this recipe, the chicken needs to marinate for an hour or so before cooking, so make sure you allow extra time for this. If you are using wooden skewers, you'll need to soak them in water for a minimum of 10 minutes before use so they don't burn during cooking. Alternatively, get yourself a set of stainless steel skewers – there's no need for soaking and it's easier to thread on the ingredients.

Serves 4

500 g chicken thigh fillets, trimmed and cut into large
    bite-sized pieces
olive or canola oil, for grilling
1 green or red capsicum, seeds and membrane removed,
    cut into bite-sized pieces

Marinade
2 tablespoons canola oil
½ garlic clove, minced
juice of 1 lemon
½ brown onion, roughly chopped
½ cup flat-leaf parsley leaves
pinch of sea salt and freshly ground black pepper

Israeli salad
2 tomatoes, chopped
1 continental cucumber, chopped

2 tablespoons finely chopped flat-leaf parsley

1 teaspoon lemon juice

pinch of sea salt

1 tablespoon olive oil

1. To make the marinade, place all the ingredients in a blender and blitz until well combined. The consistency will be quite thick.

2. Scoop the marinade into a zip-lock bag or large bowl, add the chicken and turn to coat well. Place in the fridge to marinate for 1 hour.

3. Meanwhile, prepare the salad. Place all the ingredients in a bowl and gently toss to combine.

4. Preheat a hot grill plate or chargrill pan over medium heat and lightly grease with olive or canola oil.

5. Wipe off any excess marinade from the chicken pieces and thread evenly onto four skewers, alternating with the capsicum.

6. Add to the grill and cook, turning every couple of minutes, for about 10 minutes or until the chicken is cooked through. The exact cooking time will depend on the size of the chicken pieces.

7. Serve the skewers with the accompanying salad.

VEGETABLE COTTAGE PIES

Red split lentils are quick and easy to use and, unlike the majority of legumes, they don't need to be presoaked. As their skins have been removed, they split naturally into two halves and cook very quickly.

Makes 8

3 tablespoons olive oil
1 brown onion, finely chopped
1 leek, white part only, washed and finely chopped
3 carrots, finely chopped
3 sticks celery, finely chopped
1 large sweet potato, peeled and finely chopped
375 g red split lentils
2½ cups (300 g) frozen peas
3 tablespoons tomato paste
3 cups (750 ml) vegetable stock
pinch of sea salt and freshly ground black pepper
8 sheets filo pastry, thawed

1. Preheat the oven to 180°C and line a baking tray with baking paper.
2. Heat the olive oil in a large deep frying pan or saucepan over medium heat. Add the onion, leek, carrot, celery and sweet potato and cook, stirring, for 10 minutes or until softened.

3. Stir in the lentils, peas and tomato paste, add the stock and season with salt and pepper. Reduce the heat to low and cook for 10 minutes, stirring regularly. Keep an eye on the lentils as you don't want them to go mushy. Remove from heat.

4. Using one sheet of filo pastry per pie, first fold the pastry to create a double layer, and then scoop 2 tablespoons of the pie filling evenly along the pastry. Fold in the sides and roll so that it looks like a cigar shape. You don't want to add too much filling as it will split the pastry when you fold it in.

5. Place on the prepared baking tray. Repeat with the remaining pastry and filling to make eight pies. If you have leftover filling, you can make additional pies by repeating the process above with more filo pastry.

6. Bake for 20 minutes or until the pastry is golden and the filling is hot.

SALLY'S VEGETABLE RISOTTO

My wife is a great cook, and even though I'm not a huge fan of risotto I love this version. A traditional risotto is quite creamy, with butter and cheese as key ingredients; however, this one is wonderfully flavoursome without those elements, making it a great addition to your IWL eating plan.

There's no need to limit yourself to the vegetables listed here – mushrooms, sweet potato and beetroot are all popular risotto options, and you could also add some chicken if you like.

We make this in a cast-iron pot, starting on the stovetop then transferring it to the oven to complete the cook, meaning we don't have to stand there and stir for 45 minutes. Of course, you can cook it on the stovetop if you prefer, but this will require closer supervision.

Serves 4

300 g pumpkin (any variety), skin on, cut into bite-sized pieces
olive oil spray
2 tablespoons olive oil
½ brown onion, finely chopped
2 garlic cloves, finely chopped
1 cup (200 g) arborio rice
2 cups (500 ml) vegetable stock
1 head broccoli, cut into florets, stalk chopped
2 large handfuls of kale leaves, stalks removed

1. Preheat the oven to 200°C.
2. Spread out the pumpkin on a baking tray and spray with olive oil. Roast for 25 minutes or until tender and lightly golden on the edges.
3. Heat the olive oil in a large flameproof casserole dish over medium heat. Add the onion and garlic and cook until softened and lightly coloured.
5. Add the cooked pumpkin, rice, stock, broccoli and kale. Mix well.
6. Cover and place in the oven. It should take about 40 minutes to cook.

KIMCHI PANCAKE

This is a very popular dish in Korea. Kimchi is a fermented food – most commonly made with cabbage that is fermented with salt and seasonings, including chilli, garlic and ginger. During the fermentation process, good bacteria convert carbohydrate into lactic acid, which preserves the vegetables and gives them their tangy taste. This is a 'gut-friendly' food that has seen a rise in popularity in Western countries due to the recent interest in gut health, and it is readily available in larger supermarkets and Asian grocery stores. Fermented vegetables are a wonderful addition to your eating plan, but all vegetables and wholegrain carbohydrates will improve your gut health.

Serves 4

2 cups (400 g) chopped kimchi (cabbage variety)
½ cup kimchi juice and water (use the juice from the container the kimchi comes in topped up with water)
1 teaspoon sea salt
1 teaspoon sugar (any variety)
1 handful of beansprouts
1 cup (160 g) plain or self-raising wholemeal flour
olive oil spray

1. Place all the ingredients (except the olive oil spray) and ½ cup (125 ml) water in a large bowl and mix together well.
2. Heat a large frying pan over low heat and spray with olive oil.
3. Pour half the mixture into the pan and cook for 2 minutes or until the bottom of the pancake sets and is easy to flip.
4. Flip the pancake over and cook the other side for 1 minute or until set and lightly golden.
5. Slide the pancake onto a plate and cover to keep warm.
6. Repeat with the remaining mixture to make a second pancake. Cut each pancake in half to serve four people.

SALLY'S FRIED RICE

The secret ingredients here are tamarind paste and kecap manis, both of which you can buy from larger supermarkets. Don't stress if you can't find one or both – it'll still be delicious. When we cook rice in our house, we normally make 2–3 cups (which yields 4–5 cups when cooked) and freeze the leftovers to have ready for a speedy weeknight dinner. Make sure to freeze any leftovers within 3 minutes of cooking.

Like most of the IWL recipes, you can personalise this one to suit your tastes and what you've got on hand. Nobody should be running to the shops to buy a green capsicum if they have a red one in the fridge! If you prefer, you can use a packet of frozen stir-fry vegetables – it'll save you chopping time too.

Serves 8

1 cup (200 g) brown rice
olive or sesame oil, for pan-frying
3 garlic cloves, finely chopped
2 spring onions, finely chopped, using green leaf
6 cups variety of vegetables (for example, a combination of
carrots, broccoli, green beans, capsicum, baby corn, water
chestnuts, kale/baby spinach/rocket, kaleslaw, cabbage), cut
into bite-sized pieces
2–3 tablespoons tamarind paste
2–3 tablespoons soy sauce
2 tablespoons kecap manis
sesame seeds or fried shallots, to serve

1. Cook the rice according to the packet instructions (see also Tip) and set aside.
2. Heat a drizzle of olive or sesame oil in a large frying pan or wok over medium heat. Add the garlic and cook until softened and fragrant.
3. Add the hardest vegetables to the pan first and cook until tender, then add the softer vegetables (excluding any leafy greens, which take very little time to cook) and cook until tender.
4. Add the cooked rice and toss it through the vegetables.
5. Stir in the leafy greens, tamarind, soy sauce and kecap manis.
6. Stir to combine, then remove from the heat. Serve garnished with sesame seeds or fried shallots.

Tip: The absorption method is a simple way to cook rice. This method requires 1½ cups (375 ml) water for every 1 cup (200 g) uncooked rice. Combine the rice and water in a saucepan and bring to the boil, stirring occasionally. Reduce the heat to low, then cover and simmer, stirring occasionally, for 12–15 minutes or until tender. Fluff up the rice with a fork and serve.

EGGPLANT AND TOFU MISO NOODLES

Many people cringe when they realise tofu is on the menu. However, it's an extremely nutritious food that is high in protein and a good source of calcium. It's also very tasty, when cooked correctly. Pan-fried tofu is a delicious addition to many dishes, in place of meat.

Serves 4

400 g wholegrain noodles (any variety is fine)
olive oil, for cooking
225 g firm tofu, cut into bite-sized pieces (see Fun fact)
1 large eggplant, cut into bite-sized cubes
1 head broccoli, cut into florets
3 large handfuls of dark green leafy vegetables (kale, baby
    spinach leaves or rocket)
1 tablespoon sesame seeds

Miso sauce
⅔ cup (160 ml) vegetable stock
2 tablespoons white or yellow miso paste
2 tablespoons honey
2 garlic cloves, crushed
1 teaspoon grated ginger

1. To make the sauce, combine all the ingredients in a bowl.
   Set aside.

2. Cook the noodles according to the packet instructions.

3. Heat a splash of olive oil in a frying pan over high heat. Add the tofu and cook for 30 seconds, then stir and leave for another 30 seconds. Remove from the pan.

4. Add a little more oil if necessary, then add the eggplant and broccoli and about one-quarter of the sauce. Cook, stirring regularly, still over the same heat, for about 10 minutes or until the eggplant is tender.

5. Add the noodles, tofu and remaining sauce to the pan and mix through. Throw in the leafy greens.

6. Sprinkle with the sesame seeds and serve hot.

Fun fact: Tofu is made by curdling soy milk made from soy beans and pressing the curds into blocks – similar to the way cheese is made from milk. It comes in different varieties with different levels of firmness. The two main kinds are silken and regular. Silken has a softer consistency than regular tofu and each one suits different types of dishes. This recipe works best with a firm regular tofu. Try them all and find one that you like best.

EDAMAME FALAFELS WITH GREEK YOGHURT OR HUMMUS

Falafel is a traditional Middle Eastern food. They are typically made with chickpeas and deep-fried. But they are also delicious when made with fava beans, specifically broad beans, or edamame, as used in this recipe. Better still, they don't need to be deep-fried and can be baked in the oven, making a much healthier dish. They are delicious when paired with hummus or Greek yoghurt, and make great snacks or meals when entertaining guests.

For this recipe, you have the option to use either dried chickpeas or the tinned variety. If using dried, you will need to soak the chickpeas overnight, so start this recipe the day before.

Serves 4

200 g frozen edamame, shelled, or 200 g broad beans, frozen,
    pre-shelled
sea salt and freshly ground black pepper
1 cup (200 g) dried chickpeas, soaked in water overnight,
    drained, or 1 x 400 g tinned chickpeas, drained and rinsed
½ cup coriander leaves
3 tablespoons flat-leaf parsley leaves
2 garlic cloves, crushed
1 tablespoon ground cumin
1 red chilli, finely chopped
1 teaspoon finely grated lemon zest

2 tablespoons wholemeal flour

1 egg, lightly whisked

½ cup (140 g) Greek yoghurt or hummus (see page 237)

1. Preheat the oven to 180°C and line a baking tray with baking paper.
2. Boil the edamame or broad beans and a pinch of salt for 1 minute. Drain.
3. Place the edamame, chickpeas, coriander, parsley, garlic, cumin, chilli, lemon zest, egg, flour and a pinch of salt and pepper in a bowl. Mix until well combined.
4. Form heaped tablespoons of the mixture into small patties.
5. Place the falafels on the prepared baking tray and bake for 20 minutes.
6. Serve hot with Greek yoghurt or hummus.

SNACKS AND SIDES

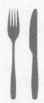

RUSTIC HUMMUS

Legumes, such as beans, peas, lentils, peanuts and chickpeas, are a handy ingredient to have in your pantry. They are cheap, a great source of plant protein, and can be used in a wide variety of dishes. This Middle Eastern dip allows the chickpeas to shine, and with the unusual addition of capers and egg, this is a recipe you will find hard to resist making all the time.

Makes 1½ cups

400 g tinned chickpeas, drained and rinsed
2 tablespoons tahini
2 garlic cloves, crushed
juice of ½ large lemon
1 egg
1 tablespoon capers
sea salt and freshly ground black pepper

1. Half-fill a small saucepan with water and bring to the boil.
2. Meanwhile, place the chickpeas, tahini, garlic and lemon juice in a food processor and blend until smooth. Scoop the mixture into a large bowl that is suitable for storage.
3. Add a pinch of salt to the boiling water. Using a spoon, gently dip the egg in and out of the boiling water, then lower it into the water. This will prevent the shell from cracking. Cook for 7 minutes, then remove and cool under cold water. Peel the egg and finely chop, then add to the hummus mixture.

4. Add the capers and a pinch of pepper to the hummus. Mix together with a fork.

5. Serve immediately or cover and store in the fridge for up to 2 weeks.

Fun fact: Did you know that a food is considered a legume if it has seeds inside its pods and only the seeds are eaten? Where we eat both the seed and the pod (for example, green beans and snow peas) it is considered to be a vegetable.

ROAST BUTTERNUT PUMPKIN HUMMUS

Another variation on traditional hummus, the butternut pumpkin adds an earthy, rich and sweet flavour to this recipe. This delicious dip goes well with toasted wholegrain bread, torn pieces of wholemeal Lebanese bread, or with sticks of raw vegetables.

Makes 2 cups

400 g butternut pumpkin, peeled and cut into large chunks
2 garlic cloves, peeled, chopped
¼ cup (60 ml) olive oil
1 x 400 g can chickpeas, drained and rinsed
½ tablespoon tahini
juice of 1 lemon
sea salt and freshly ground black pepper

1. Preheat the oven to 160°C and line a baking tray with baking paper.
2. Place the pumpkin in a large bowl, add the garlic and 2 tablespoons olive oil and mix to coat well.
3. Spread the pumpkin over the prepared baking tray in a single layer and bake for 25 minutes or until tender. Keep an eye on it – you don't want the pumpkin to colour. Remove and set aside to cool.

4. Place the pumpkin, garlic, chickpeas, tahini, lemon juice, remaining olive oil and ¼ cup (60 ml) water in a food processor. Season with salt and pepper and pulse until smooth and well combined.

5. Serve immediately or scoop into sealed containers or jars and refrigerate. The hummus will keep in the fridge for 2 weeks.

WHOLE ROAST CAULIFLOWER WITH LEMON AND CHILLI

Just like broccoli, cauliflower is a cruciferous vegetable that is packed full of antioxidants that protect the body against damage. On its own it can be a little boring, but it's a whole new ballgame if you cook it creatively. Give this recipe a go to reinvigorate your desire for this nutritious vegetable.

Serves 4

1 head cauliflower
olive oil, for drizzling
finely grated zest and juice of ½ lemon
dried chilli flakes, for sprinkling
sea salt and freshly ground black pepper

1. Preheat the oven to 180°C. Pre-line a baking tray with baking paper.
2. Place the whole cauliflower in a large saucepan of water. Bring to the boil, then reduce the heat and simmer for 7 minutes. Drain.
3. Cut off the stalk and remove the leaves. Place in the baking tray.
4. Scatter the lemon zest over the cauliflower, then pour over the lemon juice and a drizzle of olive oil. Sprinkle lightly with chilli flakes, season with salt and pepper, and roast for 35 minutes or until tender and lightly golden. Cut into wedges and serve.

BASIL PESTO

Basil is not a difficult herb to grow – it just needs plenty of sun and plenty of water, otherwise it quickly turns to seed. It's a great choice as it's very expensive to buy and often we only use a little and see the rest go to waste. There is no better feeling than having organic produce at your fingertips, and whenever there's an abundance you can make delicious, nutritious recipes like this.

If you have one, use a mortar and pestle when making this recipe – it gives a great rustic finish and taste, and it's a really fun way to make it.

Makes 2 cups

½ cup (80 g) pine nuts (walnuts are also good here)
4 garlic cloves, roughly chopped
½ teaspoon sea salt
½ teaspoon dried chilli flakes
3 cups basil leaves
½ cup (40 g) grated parmesan
3 tablespoons extra virgin olive oil

1. Tip the pine nuts into a dry frying pan and toast over medium heat, stirring frequently, for 2–3 minutes or until golden. Keep an eye on them as they can burn easily. Set aside to cool.

2. Using a large mortar and pestle or a food processor, pound or process the garlic, salt and chilli to form a paste.

3. Add the basil and pound or process until a puree forms.

4. Add the pine nuts and pound or pulse just until they break up a bit (you want a bit of texture here).

5. Add the parmesan and olive oil and combine well.

6. Serve immediately or scoop into a sealed container or jar and refrigerate. The pesto will keep in the fridge for up to 2 weeks.

PEA PESTO

This is another great dip to make and have on hand in the fridge for when you feel hungry. It is delicious served with wholegrain Lebanese bread and is another great dish to have when entertaining guests.

As with the basil pesto recipe, this can also be made with a mortar and pestle.

Makes 1 cup

⅓ cup (50 g) pine nuts
1 cup (120 g) frozen peas, thawed
2 tablespoons olive oil
3 tablespoons grated parmesan
1 teaspoon finely chopped basil
sea salt and freshly ground black pepper

1. Tip the pine nuts into a dry frying pan and toast over medium heat, stirring frequently, for 2–3 minutes or until golden. Keep an eye on them as they can burn easily. Set aside to cool.
2. Using a large mortar and pestle or a food processor, add the pine nuts to the other ingredients and pulse until well combined but with a little texture remaining.
3. Serve immediately, or scoop into a sealed container or jar and refrigerate. The pesto will keep in the fridge for up to 10 days.

KALE CHIPS

Kale is a wonderful vegetable to grow in your garden. It's a nutritious addition to the vegetables on your plate and also makes a great snack when roasted into chips. I don't offer any quantities here as it's more of a process than a recipe. Make as many or as few chips as you like.

freshly picked kale leaves, thick stems removed
olive oil spray
dried chilli flakes
roasted garlic flakes
dried parsley
sea salt

1. Preheat the oven to 180°C and line a large baking tray (or as many trays as you need) with baking paper.
2. Tear the kale leaves into large bite-sized pieces and spray with olive oil. Spread out in a single layer on the prepared tray.
3. Mix together the chilli flakes, roasted garlic flakes, dried parsley and a good pinch of salt. Sprinkle this mixture over the kale leaves – it will stick to the olive oil and form a delicious coating on the kale.
4. Bake for 5 minutes or until crisp and lightly coloured around the edges.
5. These are best served warm from the oven rather than being kept for a later snack.

SAUERKRAUT

Cabbages are an easy vegetable to grow at home, so if you have the space I would strongly recommend it. A little bit of water in some good nutrient-rich soil and they will grow with ease. Their protective outer leaves mean they are also very resistant to bugs so there won't be a need for pesticides.

Makes 2 cups

2 cabbages
3 tablespoons table salt

1. Remove the outer leaves from the cabbages and wash thoroughly. Make sure your hands and everything that comes into contact with the cabbage are clean and sterile (see Tips).
2. Slice each cabbage in half and remove the white core.
3. Chop into thin strips and place in a large bowl with the salt.
4. Using your hands, rub the salt into the cabbage, massaging until you have a much-reduced volume of cabbage sitting in its own brine. This will take 5–10 minutes.
5. Add the cabbage and brine to a sterilised jar, making sure the brine covers the cabbage completely. Add some water if the cabbage is not covered.
6. Seal the jar and leave in a cool, dark environment for up to 2 weeks. The longer you leave it the sourer the flavour will become, but make sure you keep an eye on it regularly to ensure it doesn't dry out.
7. Once opened, store the jar in the fridge for up to 2 weeks.

Tips: Sauerkraut can be made in large batches. We often grow up to a dozen cabbages at one time, harvest them all together and use them for sauerkraut. A jar of sauerkraut makes for a great family gift.

This is a fun recipe to make with the kids on the weekend. Just make sure everything is sterile! To sterilise jars and equipment, I prefer to use the stovetop. Add the jars and lids to a deep saucepan of cold water. Turn heat to high and bring to the boil. Reduce heat and boil for 10 minutes. Line a tray with paper towel and carefully remove the jars from the water. After cooling, pat dry with paper towel.

SWEET TREATS

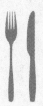

BANANA AND CHOCOLATE BLISS BALLS

Bliss balls, protein balls, energy balls . . . whatever you call them, they are certainly the latest food trend sweeping the health and wellness scene. But there's no denying they can be a wonderfully filling and wholesome snack, giving you the sweet hit you're after. It's much better to reach for one of these than devour a block of chocolate or a packet of biscuits to get over that mid-afternoon hump, so make a batch on the weekend and keep them in the fridge for up to 2 weeks. Just be careful not to eat them all in one go. Divide them into containers or wrap them into portions to help with self-control.

Makes 20

2 large bananas
2¼ cups (200 g) rolled oats
1 egg
2 tablespoons olive oil
3 tablespoons natural peanut butter (100% peanuts)
1 teaspoon vanilla extract
150 g dark chocolate, chopped

1. Preheat the oven to 170°C and line a large baking tray with baking paper.
2. Mash the bananas in a large bowl, then add the remaining ingredients and mix well.
3. Form tablespoons of the mixture into balls.
4. Place the balls on the prepared baking tray and bake for 18 minutes. Serve warm or cold.

FLOURLESS ALMOND AND ORANGE CAKE

In this recipe whole oranges are cooked and then puréed – skin, pips and all. Not only is this cake incredibly moreish and moist, it is also nutritious and a wonderful treat that guests will love.

Makes 1 cake

2 oranges, tops removed
6 eggs
1 teaspoon baking powder
1 cup (360 g) honey
2½ cups (400 g) almonds, plus extra small handful (30 g) for the
   crust

1. Preheat the oven to 160°C and line a 20 cm round cake tin with two layers of baking paper.
2. Using a sharp knife, stab holes in the oranges to pierce them all over.
3. Place the oranges in a large microwave-safe bowl and pour in enough water to come one-third of the way up the side of the oranges. Cook on high for 5 minutes. Set aside to cool.
4. Crack the eggs into a bowl and beat with electric beaters to the consistency of lightly whipped cream, adding the baking powder and honey halfway through the blending process – when the eggs start to foam.
5. Place the almonds in a blender and pulse to a flour consistency. Fold the almond meal into the egg mixture using a wooden spoon.

6. Cut the oranges into quarters and blitz to a puree in the blender. Fold into the cake batter until well combined.

7. Pour the batter into the prepared tin and bake for 30 minutes.

8. Using a mortar and pestle, lightly grind the extra almonds to a rubble. Sprinkle the almonds over the partially cooked cake and return to the oven.

9. Bake for a further 20–30 minutes. Start checking after 20 minutes as everybody's oven is different. The cake is cooked when you can insert a knife or skewer in the centre and it comes out with just a couple of crumbs clinging to it. If it is still sticky, put it back in the oven for a few more minutes, then check again.

10. Cool in the tin for 20 minutes, then carefully turn out and enjoy.

DATE AND ALMOND COOKIES

These cookies are great to make in larger batches when hosting a party. They also make for great snacks when you want to add a little variety to your weekly IWL meal plan. Adding variety to your diet will ensure you don't get sick of the foods you are eating and enable you to stick to the plan lifelong.

Makes 10

1 cup (160 g) almonds
3 tablespoons fresh dates, pitted
1 tablespoon maple syrup
4 drops vanilla essence
¼ teaspoon ground cinnamon
3 tablespoons rolled oats

1. Preheat the oven to 160°C and line a large baking tray with baking paper.
2. Place the almonds in a food processor until ground to flour consistency. Add the other ingredients and blend until smooth. If the mixture is struggling to mix, add 1–2 teaspoons water.
3. Roll tablespoons of the mixture into balls and place on the prepared baking tray. Press down on each ball with the back of a spoon to flatten slightly.
4. Bake for 10 minutes. Remove and allow to cool completely on the tray or on a wire rack. Store in an airtight container in the fridge for up to 10 days.

ACKNOWLEDGEMENTS

I'd like to thank the community of people who have written to me since the release of my first book, *Interval Weight Loss*. This has inspired me to continue spreading this important message and to give those following the Interval Weight Loss plan more information and support to ensure they succeed.

To my wife, Sally. Thank you for being the best, for always being there for me, and for helping me shape this book and message. I am very lucky to have such an intelligent and beautiful person in my life. I love you very much.

To my mother, Diane, and my brother, Andrew. Thank you for all your love, support and generosity. I am eternally grateful for all that you do and all that you have

255

given, and blessed to have such a wonderful, caring and kind-hearted family.

To my friends who have helped with this book. Particular mention to my close friends Ed White, Matthew Mooney, Kris Klein and Chris Wilkins. I very much enjoyed our sessions bouncing around ideas on *Interval Weight Loss* over a run, surf and pizza. I am very grateful for all the help you provided and truly value your friendships.

To my publisher, Penguin Random House. This is, of course, not possible without your support and belief in me. And to my commissioning editor at Penguin Random House, Sophie Ambrose. I thoroughly enjoy working with you and am extremely grateful for your expertise and professionalism in assisting me to translate this message to the population.

WEIGHT-LOSS TEMPLATE

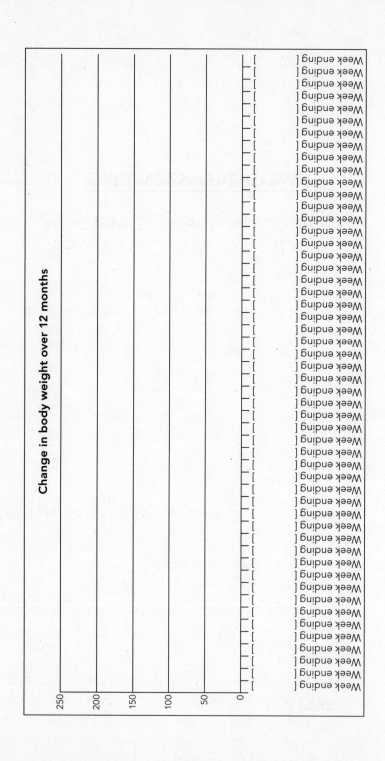

Change in body weight over 12 months

250

200

150

100

50

0

Week ending [   ]
Week ending [   ]
Week ending [   ]
Week ending [   ]
Week ending [   ]
Week ending [   ]
Week ending [   ]
Week ending [   ]
Week ending [   ]
Week ending [   ]
Week ending [   ]
Week ending [   ]
Week ending [   ]
Week ending [   ]
Week ending [   ]
Week ending [   ]
Week ending [   ]
Week ending [   ]
Week ending [   ]
Week ending [   ]
Week ending [   ]
Week ending [   ]
Week ending [   ]
Week ending [   ]
Week ending [   ]
Week ending [   ]
Week ending [   ]
Week ending [   ]
Week ending [   ]
Week ending [   ]
Week ending [   ]
Week ending [   ]
Week ending [   ]
Week ending [   ]
Week ending [   ]
Week ending [   ]
Week ending [   ]
Week ending [   ]
Week ending [   ]
Week ending [   ]
Week ending [   ]
Week ending [   ]

THE DO'S AND DON'TS OF INTERVAL WEIGHT LOSS

Write this list on a piece of paper and keep it on your fridge.

The do's

- Include a source of wholegrain carbs with every meal.
- Eat before going grocery shopping.
- Eat away from technological distraction.
- Change your exercise routine every second month.
- Do the things on your 'to do' list that you most dislike first.
- Aim for approximately 2 kilograms weight loss every second month.

- Weigh yourself on the same day and time each week.
- Weigh yourself weekly and plot the weight to analyse the trend.
- Record your body weight so you can visually monitor it.
- Eat five meals per day.
- Write a 'to do' list.
- Plan each day the night before, or first thing in the morning.
- Cook extra food to save for leftovers the next day.
- Drink a glass of water before every meal or when you feel hungry.
- Wear an activity monitoring device every day and record your movement.

The don'ts

- Under no circumstances continue with weight loss during a weight-maintenance month.
- Do not weigh yourself every day.
- Don't eliminate wholegrain carbohydrates from a meal just because you see an increase on the scales.
- Don't change your weight-loss goal just because it seems easy and you want to reach your end goal faster.
- Don't give up if you don't see weight loss when you first start the IWL plan – read the book again as

there may be a couple of things you need to tweak in your lifestyle.

- Don't just write your body weight down on a piece of scrap paper and tell yourself you will remember it – plot it on a graph and monitor the trend over time.

Last but not least

- Read this book more than once – the more times you read it, the more you will pick up.
- Message us and update us with your progress and questions at the 'Dr Nick Fuller's Interval Weight Loss' Facebook page.
- Take the opportunity to ask all your questions at the Dr Nick Fuller Facebook live events.
- Follow us on Instagram @intervalweightloss.
- Subscribe to our free e-newsletter at: www.intervalweightloss.com.au.

FOODS YOU CAN EAT
WHEN HUNGRY

Write down this list on a piece of paper and keep it on your fridge.

Nuts
Seeds
Dips (see some suggestions in Snacks and Sides)
Carrot and celery sticks
Oven-roasted vegetables – any type
Fruit
No-fat flavoured or plain yoghurt
Boiled egg
Wholegrain toast with 100 per cent nut spread, avocado,
    or 100 per cent fruit spread
Blueberries/raspberries with yoghurt

HUNGER SCALE

This is a handy tool to use each meal time until you gain a full appreciation for your hunger cues

-1	0	1	2	3	4
Full and uncomfortable	Not at all hungry	Satisfied	Slightly hungry	Somewhat hungry	Hungry

STORE CUPBOARD ESSENTIALS

Keep a good supply of the following foods in your kitchen, and when they start to run low make sure you add them to your shopping list before they run out completely. Don't be overwhelmed by this list as these are staples that last for a long time, and for those who are beginners or have no cooking skills at all, they can be accumulated gradually, as your confidence with cooking develops. If you don't like a certain food or can't find it, there's no need to buy it – just substitute it with another healthy favourite.

Dried herbs and spices: black pepper, oregano, chilli flakes, coriander, basil, thyme, turmeric, cumin, mixed herbs, mustard seeds

Oils: olive or canola oil

Dried goods: unsalted dry-roasted or raw nuts, variety of seeds (e.g. sunflower, flaxseed, pumpkin, sesame), wholemeal flour (plain and self-raising), dried breadcrumbs, various types of pasta (including wholemeal), rice (basmati, brown), rolled oats, couscous, pearl barley, quinoa, dried pulses (lentils, chickpeas, black beans, split peas), sugar

Tinned food: tomatoes, chickpeas, lentils, red kidney beans, black beans, lima beans, three-bean mix, corn, beetroot, pineapple, fish (tuna or salmon in spring water or olive oil), tomato paste (low salt)

Condiments: soy sauce, ready-made vegetable stock, honey, lemon juice, lime juice, maple syrup, tahini paste (hulled or unhulled), nut butter, jarred garlic, ginger and chilli (all-natural jarred with vinegar only, and as a back-up only to fresh sources)

Long-lasting vegetables: onions, sweet potato, ginger, garlic, potato, pumpkin

Perishables: milk, no-fat or low-fat yoghurt (no added sugar), eggs, wholegrain bread

Frozen food: blueberries, mixed berries, edamame beans, frozen vegetables

Beverages: green tea, variety of herbal teas, coffee

RECIPE INDEX